T5-BPZ-141

HEALTH CARE POLICY IN THE UNITED STATES

edited by

JOHN G. BRUHN
PENNSYLVANIA STATE
UNIVERSITY-HARRISBURG

A GARLAND SERIES

Health Care Policy in the United States
John G. Bruhn, editor

MEDICAID AND THE COSTS OF FEDERALISM, 1984–1992

JEAN DONOVAN GILMAN

GARLAND PUBLISHING, Inc.
A MEMBER OF THE TAYLOR & FRANCIS GROUP
NEW YORK & LONDON / 1998

Library of Congress Cataloging-in-Publication Data

Gilman, Jean Donovan.
  Medicaid and the costs of federalism, 1984–1992 / Jean
Donovan Gilman.
      p.   cm. — (Health care policy in the United States)
  Includes bibliographical references and index.
  ISBN 0-8153-3278-5 (alk. paper)
  1. Medicaid—History. 2. Medicaid—Finance. 3. Intergov-
ernmental fiscal relations—United States. I. Title. II. Series:
Health care policy in the United States (New York, N.Y.)
RA412.4.G55 1998
368.4'2'00973—dc21

                                                    98-47361

Printed on acid-free, 250-year-life paper
Manufactured in the United States of America

This book is dedicated to my children, Ian and Caitrin.

Contents

Acknowledgements

My children Ian and Caitrin have provided both the greatest inspiration and the greatest obstacles to the completion of this book. Their confidence in my ability to succeed in this endeavor, which they did not fully comprehend, was at once humbling and motivating. Yet their mere presence continually drew me away from this task.

As with all difficult endeavors in life, numerous people were instrumental in helping me along the way. Jim Gilman demonstrated his support in many important ways—not the least of which was caring for our children so lovingly. To the extent this book reflects clarity of thought and readable prose, Martha Derthick, my mentor at the University of Virginia, deserves the credit. And where it does not, I assume responsibility for ignoring her good advice. Had she not displayed an uncommon commitment to me, this book would never have been completed.

A special group of colleagues at Mary Baldwin College kept me focused on the meaning of life, supplying me with timely encouragement, advice, flowers, notes, and sympathetic ears (Judy, Carrie, Anne, Mary Hill, John, Brian, Kathleen, Alan, Marlena, Laura, Roussie, Nan, Dinah, Paul, Lydia, Edward, Lallon, Rod, and many others). The Dean of the College, James Lott, also gave me vital support and assistance. I want to thank each of these and my many friends and family, who never lost confidence in me (or at least never expressed it), helping to sustain my own wavering optimism and pushing me on to the end. And finally, I am indebted to Rebecca

Wipfler, my editor at Garland Publishing, for her invaluable assistance at the last stages of the publication process.

Abbreviations

ACIR	Advisory Commission on Intergovernmental Relations
ADC	Aid to Dependent Children
AFDC	Aid to Families of Dependent Children
AHCPR	Agency for Health Care Policy and Research
CBO	Congressional Budget Office
C&N	*Congress and the Nation*
CQWR	*Congressional Quarterly Weekly Report*
CQA	*Congressional Quarterly Almanac*
DHEW	Department of Health, Education and Welfare
DHHS	Department of Health and Human Services
DMS	Division of Medical Services
DSH	Disproportionate Share Hospital
EPSDTP	Early and Periodic Screening, Diagnosis and Treatment Program
ESRD	End Stage Renal Disease
FICA	Federal Insurance Contributions Act
FY	Fiscal Year
GAO	General Accounting Office
GRH	Gramm-Rudman-Hollings (Balanced Budget and Emergency Deficit Control Act of 1985)
HCFA	Health Care Financing Administration
HECC	House Energy and Commerce Committee
HEW	Department of Health, Education and Welfare
HHS	Department of Health and Human Services
HI	Hospital Insurance (Medicare Part A)
HMO	Health Maintenance Organization
HWMC	House Ways and Means Committee

ICF	Intermediate Care Facility
MSA	Medical Services Administration
NGA	National Governors' Association
NYT	*New York Times*
OASDI	Old Age, Survivors, and Disability Insurance
PPS	Prospective Payment System
PRO	Peer Review Organization
PSRO	Professional Standards Review Organization
RBRVS	Resource Based Relative Value Scale
QMB	Qualified Medicare Beneficiary
SFC	Senate Finance Committee
SMI	Supplementary Medical Insurance (Medicare Part B)
SSA	Social Security Amendments
WP	*Washington Post*

Medicaid and the Costs of Federalism, 1984–1992

Introduction

CHAPTER ONE

The Explosion in Medicaid Expenditures

Rapid growth in health care expenditures has plagued this nation since 1965 when Congress first created medicare (health care insurance for the elderly) and medicaid (health care assistance for the poor). These two programs have not grown at the same rate, however. Largely owing to more favorable congressional treatment, medicare's expenditures had generally grown more rapidly than medicaid's until the late 1980s. At that time, medicaid's costs began skyrocketing, averaging 28 percent rate of growth between 1989 and 1992. This rapid growth rate represented an increase in medicaid's expenditures from $58 billion to $113 billion over those three years (Coughlin et al. 1994a, 15). Meanwhile, the annual rate of growth of medicare and private health insurance leveled off to an average of 10.7 percent and 7.2 percent respectively for the same years (Wade and Berg 1995, 11). (See Figure 1.1 for a comparison of growth in expenditures among these three health care financing approaches; and See Figure 1.2 for a comparison of growth rates.) Given the previous history of medicaid, and the impact of its sudden growth on state and federal budgets,[1] this surprising change in program expenditures invites investigation.

A number of public and private organizations have analyzed medicaid's growth over such a short time. These include: the Kaiser Commission on the Future of Medicaid, the Urban Institute, the Congressional Research Service, and the Congressional Budget Office (Buck and Klemm 1992; Coughlin et al. 1994a, CBO 1992, Merlis 1991, Rowland et al. 1993, Wade and Berg 1995). Not surprisingly,

Figure 1.1: Growth in Medicare, Medicaid, and Private Health Insurance Expenditures: 1987-1991 (in billions of dollars)

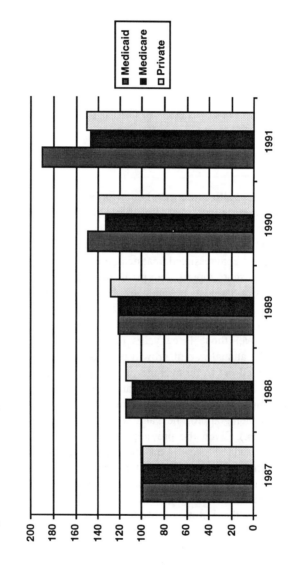

Source: Buck, Jeffrey A. And John Klemm. 1992. "Recent Trends in Medicaid Expenditures" *Health Care Financing Review, Annual Supplement*, 275.

Figure 1.2: Annual Rate of Growth in Medicare, Medicaid, and Personal Health Care Expenditures: 1987 - 1992[1]

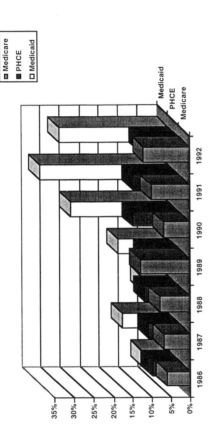

[1] Personal Health Care Expenditures (PHCE) include: all purchased services and products that are associated with individual health care, such as hospital, physician, and dental services, nursing home care, drugs, and medical supplies. It excludes expenditures for construction, program administration, government public activities, and research.

Source: U.S. Department of Health and Human Services. 1995. *Health Care Financing Review, Medicare and Medicaid Statistical Supplement,* 17.

given the complexity of the program, different institutional perspectives of researchers, and limitations in available data, conclusions about the relative impact of various causes of the growth differ somewhat. However, researchers agree that many factors contributed to medicaid's growth, including: inflation, the recession of 1990, advances in medical technology, an increase in the population, and worsening problems associated with poverty that affect the use of medical resources (drug abuse, AIDS, violence).

In addition to these, however, government sponsored enlargements in the program have emerged as a major reason for medicaid's growth. This phenomenon is most surprising in the context of medicaid's long history as the poor, little *step-sister* to the larger and more-favored medicare program. But, between the mid-1980s and the early 1990s, medicaid became the Cinderella of health care programs. It was transformed from the unpopular, over-extended, and under-appreciated program into everyone's favorite choice for expansion at both the state and national levels. From 1984 until 1990, Congress repeatedly extended the program's eligibility, services, and other features. The states also greatly enlarged the medicaid program. Beginning gradually in 1986, but then more energetically between 1990 and 1992, numerous states engaged in practices that bloated medicaid expenditures. In overlapping stages, from 1984 until 1992, first the federal government, and then the states expanded the medicaid program, contributing mightily to its growth in expenditures.

Sara Rosenbaum captures the extent of the congressional expansions in the following passage:

> Years later, it is still striking to consider how a decade that began with the election of a president who believed in reduced direct federal spending . . . could have concluded with unprecedented expansions in the most expensive of all poor people's entitlement programs. Over a six year period, beginning in 1984, more than a half million pregnant women, between four and five million children, and millions of low income elderly and disabled Medicare beneficiaries were made eligible for Medicaid. Maternity and pediatric benefits were expanded, particularly in the case of children under age 21. The Medicaid enrollment process was fundamentally restructured in order to make access to coverage easier. The statute's provider reimbursement provisions were strengthened. In short, federal

lawmakers altered virtually every feature that helps determine Medicaid's size and scope (1993a, 47).

State governments not only expanded medicaid eligibility, services, and reimbursement in response to federal mandates,[2] but they also exploited a loophole in the medicaid law enabling them to leverage billions of additional federal matching funds. Beginning in 1986, they undertook various financing schemes that increased their revenues from the federal government without incurring additional costs. These schemes greatly enlarged total medicaid expenditures. Approximately $17 billion, 26 percent of the total increase between 1988 and 1992, is attributable to the states' use of Disproportionate Share Payments (or DSP) to hospitals, one of the most common of these financing schemes (Coughlin et al. 1994a, 152). Health policy analyst Victor Miller concluded,

> much of the increase in [overall] medicaid costs in 1991 and 1992 reflected no increases in health costs but rather manipulation by state governments of the Medicaid open-ended entitlement system to generate what was essentially general revenue sharing for states (quoted in Morgan 1994b).

Prior to the mid-1980s, neither level of government had demonstrated an inclination to expand medicaid. Bent on controlling health care costs, the states and Congress had always found medicaid an easy target for cutbacks. The enlargements that occurred in the late 1980s and early 1990s were unprecedented and unexpected. This book will examine the nature and scope of the government expansions at each level, as well as the environmental, political, and institutional factors that promoted them. Furthermore, it will further answer the following questions: Why did each level of government expand the medicaid program during those years? Why was medicaid alone chosen for significant enlargement, and not another program? And finally, given the severe fiscal pressures on each level of government, how did state and federal officials manage to enlarge the program to such an unprecedented extent?

CONGRESS

The Prior Politics of Medicaid

In Congress, medicaid has never been especially popular. It certainly has never enjoyed political support equal to that of medicare (Morone 1991). Until 1984, Congress had expanded medicaid benefits only occasionally—and hardly at all for over a decade. As recently as the late 1970s, despite repeated efforts of a Democratic President and Congress to institute modest expansions, none was enacted. In the early 1980s, under the leadership of President Reagan, with a conservative national mood, Congress chose to cut back the medicaid program while protecting medicare. Then again, during the mid 1990s, when balancing the budget took priority, a Republican Congress looked to medicaid for the greatest cutbacks. In 1984, however, despite serious fiscal constraints and the same conservative administration that had earlier instituted deep medicaid cutbacks, medicaid was singled out for expansion. Congress began extending services and benefits to the poor while curtailing the program for the elderly.

Conventional thinking about medicaid politics offers little to explain this aberration. Prevailing views of health care politics hold that medicaid has less political support than medicare and is therefore more prone to cutbacks during times of fiscal constraint. Morone explains this view in the following passage:

> Welfare medicine is difficult to legislate in the United States. And unlike most other areas—where winning the legislation poses the most political difficulty—welfare medicine is even more difficult to maintain . . . When health care costs rise more quickly than general inflation, government officials face a difficult choice. They can spend relatively more on Medicaid (perhaps at the expense of a more popular constituency), or they can cut the program back. The record of the past two decades is unambiguous—officials chose the latter (1991, 282).

Under most circumstances, but especially under fiscal pressures, policymakers have chosen to protect medicare rather than medicaid because of the different constituencies of the two programs. This view implies that medicare, as the program of a more popular constituency, would remain more secure and less prone to cutbacks than medicaid.

This is indeed what happened in 1981 under Ronald Reagan, and attempts to repeat it occurred during the 104th Congress. Such a perspective does not address the phenomenon of medicaid's repeated extension by Congress during the late 1980s, however.

Health care experts have given much attention to many of the factors that have contributed to medicaid's rise in expenditures (e.g., inflation, AIDS, violence, the aging of the population, advances in medical technology), despite the fact that these are not easily amenable to change. It is surprising that the one factor that has contributed so mightily to medicaid's cost escalation, and over which government officials presumably do have control, their own behavior, has received so little attention.

Political scientists have taken no more than a superficial look at this phenomenon of medicaid's extensions, despite its sizable impact on both state and federal budgets. Ferejohn, for example, analyzes trends in social welfare spending during the 1980s, yet entirely ignores medicaid's remarkable growth. He provides a helpful framework for understanding the historic instability in medicaid's political support that explains its frequent cutbacks, but says nothing about its potential for expansion (1991). Most political analysts of the congressional enlargements have focused upon their impact on particular populations or governments—the poor, elderly, and states.

Explanation for Congressional Expansion, 1984 to 1990

A few political analysts have offered insights into why this unusual expansion occurred. Their work helps to explain how extension of health care for the poor rose on the congressional agenda during the mid 1980s, but does not adequately clarify why medicaid was the policy of choice for congressional policymakers. Furthermore, they do not shed much light on how advocates managed to overcome significant obstacles—fiscal constraints, objections of the President, and opposition from fiscal conservatives and the states—in order to achieve a track record of success over a seven year period.

The reasons offered for why medicaid emerged on the congressional agenda fall into three main categories: worsening problems, growing political support in Congress and among interest groups, and the efforts of a powerful policy entrepreneur (Cohen 1991, Kosterlitz 1989; Morgan 1994a; Sardell 1991). Deteriorating health care conditions for the poor, caused in part by earlier medicaid cutbacks, are widely recognized as an important reason for Congress's increased attention to health care financing for the poor (Sardell 1991, Cohen 1991). These same analysts place great emphasis on the effectiveness of child health advocates in uncovering and publicizing such conditions among children during the early 1980s, and in building support for an expansion in public health care financing generally. Cohen (1991) also identifies change in partisan control of Congress— which was increasingly Democratic—and its preference for more liberal policies during the mid and later 1980s, as an important factor in altering the congressional agenda from reducing public health care financing to expanding it. Another influence often mentioned is the leadership of Henry Waxman in gaining congressional support (Morgan 1994a; Kosterlitz 1989).

Some researchers have analyzed why Congress chose the medicaid program over other possible measures to expand health care financing for the poor, especially children. Schlesinger and Kronebusch argue that the congressional preference for incremental reform in health policy is part of the answer (1990). Congress might have chosen medicare, rather than medicaid, however, to incrementally extend health care benefits to the poor elderly. Yet, while Congress expanded medicaid repeatedly, it was unable to sustain even one sizable extension in medicare. In 1988 Congress enlarged medicare benefits as part of the Medicare Catastrophic Coverage Act (MCCA), but because of controversy over its financing, repealed most parts of it the following year. Those sections of the MCCA which applied to medicaid benefits, however, remained intact.

The crucial advantage that medicaid possessed over other alternatives was its shared funding.[3] This book will demonstrate how, during an era of fiscal constraints, medicaid's shared status, generally considered a disadvantage, could become an advantage. It suggests the following line of reasoning. Fiscal constraints force policymakers to seek ways to conserve expenditures. Given the political pressure on Congress to expand health care financing for the poor, members needed to choose a policy which would produce the greatest benefit to the target population at the least cost. Although medicaid fit the bill in several respects, as others have pointed out, its unique advantage was its shared financing. Because nearly half the cost of enlargements would fall on the states, this option offered particularly useful fiscal and political advantages over other alternatives.

Medicaid's shared status sheds light on why it was chosen as the preferred policy alternative. But how advocates steered this measure through the congressional minefield of the 1980s remains a puzzle. They succeeded not just once, but repeatedly over seven years. Institutional and fiscal roadblocks, such as divided government, opposition from the President and fiscal conservatives of both parties, financial constraints imposed by the Gramm-Rudman-Hollings Budget Act (1985), and unified and public appeals from the states to halt expansions might reasonably have been expected to block or impede the efforts of medicaid advocates. No other major program experienced such generous treatment by Congress during the late 1980s. Some have suggested Waxman's leadership in Congress (Morgan 1994a, Kosterlitz 1989), the efforts of other advocates, and the increasingly liberal Congress (Cohen 1991; Sardell, 1991) as important explanations for medicaid's sweeping extensions.

Few analysts have examined the important institutional developments of the 1980s that made the task of medicaid advocates easier, however. This book will argue that changes in the norms of federalism and in the congressional budget process were critical factors in the expansion of medicaid. The budget process as practiced in the 1980s was so vital to expansions, in fact, that prior to 1980, before the use of *reconciliation*, none occurred, and after 1990, when Congress altered that process, medicaid expansions came to an abrupt halt. States

STATE MEDICAID POLITICS

The mechanism whereby the states enlarged their medicaid programs is analogous to that used by Congress. It also entails cost-shifting. However, occurring at the lower level of government, it takes a completely different form. Much has been written to describe the scope and strategies of the states in exploiting the medicaid program. These studies show that thirty nine states expanded their programs in order to exploit medicaid's open-ended matching features. In many cases, they did not even extend eligibility or services for the poor while doing so (Ku and Coughlin, 1995). State maximizing of federal grants is not new, but the cost to the federal government of these schemes was unprecedented.[4] In frustration, Richard P. Kusserow, former Inspector General of the U.S. Department of Health and Human Services (DHHS) remarked sarcastically, "The Medellin drug cartel could learn a lot about money laundering from the states" (quoted in Morgan 1993a).

One of the most important factors, analysts agree, was fiscal strain. The literature on state use of federal grants also explains why this phenomenon occurred. It outlines the extent and sources of the states' economic stress between 1989 and 1992. Of these, the congressionally mandated extensions in medicaid was among the most critical (Gold 1992; Holahan et al. 1993). They suggest this program offered unique opportunities to states to increase their revenues.

While some economists argue that, in theory, open-ended matched grants are among the most efficient (Gramlich 1990), the implementation literature suggests that, in practice, instead of keeping costs low, the open-ended type of grant is particularly vulnerable to exploitation by states (Beam 1980; Derthick 1975). These authors help in understanding the incentives inherent in matching grants, such as medicaid, and the possibility for their abuse by states—especially under conditions of fiscal strain.

Nevertheless, little has been written to address the question, why didn't the federal government intervene sooner to stop this practice? Or, how did so many states manage to design, gain approval, and implement such complex, but questionable practices? This book will examine political and institutional factors at both the state and national levels that facilitated the states' use of financing schemes to maximize their medicaid matching funds. In addition to identifying developments in state governments that assisted the states, it will explore the institutional and political factors at the national level and the extent to which these influenced the behavior of state officials.

CONCLUSION

This book will summarize why and how the states and Congress enlarged the medicaid program during the 1980s and early 1990s. The history of medicaid policymaking will also be reviewed to illustrate the uniqueness of this policy of expansion, and to uncover the factors that have influenced the politics of medicaid over time. It will also explore the influence that fiscal constraints and worsening problems in the health care sector had on policymakers at both levels. Although a number of analysts have offered various explanations for why policymakers at each level pursued this expansionary strategy, this book will focus on the influence of medicaid's shared status. And it will demonstrate how this characteristic is fundamental to understanding why this traditionally unpopular program was transformed into the Cinderella of health care programs during the late 1980s and 1990s. The environmental circumstances that heightened the advantages of shared funding and the institutional factors that helped to facilitate the exploitation of this program at both levels of government during those years will be investigated.

NOTES

1. Medicaid expenditures increased from 2.4 to 6.5 percent of the federal budget from 1985 to 1995 (HWMC *Green Book* 1992, 1759) and from 8.1 to 17.1 percent of state budgets from 1987 to 1992 (Coughlin, et al. 1994a, 83).

2. Congress as well as the courts required states to enlarge their medicaid eligibility, benefits, and reimbursement, and intervened in a number of other costly ways.

3. Schlesinger and Kronebusch also mention the advantage of medicaid's shared funding in the late 1980s in explaining the choice of medicaid over other options to provide better access to prenatal care (1990, 94).

4. Martha Derthick recounts a similar instance from the late 1960s and early 1970s in which the states succeeded in exploiting grants for Social Services. She recounts how these grants grew from $345 million in 1969 to $1.69 billion in 1972 (1975, 2).

CHAPTER TWO

Politics of Medicare and Medicaid: 1965 to 1983

From the beginning, medicare has enjoyed stronger, broader, more consistent support within Congress than medicaid. Congressional loyalty to medicaid has fluctuated, producing a "support and flail syndrome"[1] in which Congress has been quite willing to take credit for benefits, but prone to abandon medicaid beneficiaries in the face of rising costs and state opposition. As a social insurance program, medicare furnishes uniform benefits to a large, well-organized constituency and appeals to widely held values in society. Medicaid, on the other hand, is a welfare program that provides health assistance to the poor, a notoriously unpopular and weak constituency. This difference in popularity was apparent even in the administrative design and funding of the two programs, and as costs mushroomed, it became increasingly evident. While no organized opposition to the medicare program arose, this was not so for medicaid. Fiscal conservatives in Congress sought to curtail the scope of the program, and the states sought greater freedom from its mandatory requirements. Because of the difference in the popularity of medicare and medicaid, Congress adopted dramatically different approaches in dealing with them between 1965 and 1983. This chapter will illustrate and offer explanations for the contrast in the congressional treatment of these two programs.

CONTRAST IN DESIGN OF MEDICARE AND MEDICAID— 1965

Differences in the congressional approach to these programs are apparent from the beginning in the way Congress laid out their administrative and financing arrangements. One of the major reasons that Congress chose to create two separate health care financing programs in 1965—one for the elderly and one for the poor—was because of the fundamental difference in popularity of these two groups. While a single health care financing program encompassing both populations would have been simpler, the lack of support for the poor meant such a proposal was never even considered at the time. Monypenny explains the rationale for federal state programs such as medicaid. He writes,

> Federal aid programs are an outcome of a loose coalition which resorts to a mixed federal state program because it is not strong enough in individual states to secure its program, and because it is not united enough to be able to achieve a wholly federal program against the opposition which a specific program would engender (1960, 14).

The medicare program was created as a national, nearly universal, program for the elderly, with uniform benefits throughout the nation. Its funding and administration were linked to the powerful and widely popular Social Security Administration, and it was considered the "darling of the politicians and the electorate" (Stevens and Stevens 1974, 115). Medicaid, by contrast, was nobody's darling. Although it served a broad range of poor and near-poor recipients,[2] it was most closely associated with welfare recipients. Rather than assigning it to the Health component of the Department of Health, Education, and Welfare (HEW), Congress designated it to be administered by the newly created Medical Services Administration, within the Division of Medical Services (DMS) of the Bureau of Family Services, a part of the Welfare Administration. This helped to assure it "would inevitably be regarded as an intrinsic part of the administrative system of federal welfare grants to the states" (Stevens and Stevens, 1974, 77).

In addition to being firmly identified with the less powerful Welfare Administration, medicaid was further handicapped by anemic funding for personnel in its first decade, which did not help it win high marks for effectiveness among Congress and the public. When medicaid was created, only 35 positions were added to the meager 23 already employed in the DMS. This paltry crew was charged with the daunting task of designing and implementing the complex medicaid program. It had to "implement poorly drafted legislation, negotiate with powerful states, and administer a budget that was soon consuming a fifth of all federal expenses in health care—a sum running into billions of dollars" (Stevens and Stevens 1974, 78). Not surprisingly, administrative problems emerged, and instead of receiving increased funding, medicaid became a lightning rod for congressional criticism. Senate hearings in 1969 and 1970 that investigated both medicare and medicaid were especially critical of medicaid's administration (Senate Finance Committee Hearings 1969, 1970). Despite a consensus in 1970 that the DMS was severely hampered by inadequate staffing, Congress only "grudgingly increased the personnel allotment" (Thompson 1981, 121).

CONTRAST IN CONGRESSIONAL TREATMENT OF MEDICARE AND MEDICAID

The difference in the popularity of the medicaid and medicare programs was evident, not only in the design and institutional arrangements of the programs, but in the treatment of their beneficiaries between 1965 and 1983. Members of Congress consistently treated beneficiaries of medicare more generously than those of medicaid. First, they freely enlarged medicare's benefits and eligibility, and then, as costs burgeoned, they expended great energy to find adequate funding for the program while protecting beneficiaries from the effect of cutbacks. Medicaid beneficiaries did not fare so well. Sizable opposition to that program's expenses emerged almost immediately after its creation. Consequently, Congress was much less generous, awarding it relatively few and minor expansions. Congress curtailed medicaid's funding to the states, decreased benefits and eligibility among that program's most vulnerable, and granted the states increased freedom to do the same. In general, Congress failed to protect medicaid beneficiaries nearly as well as those of medicare.[3] (See Figure 2.1 for a comparison of the treatment of these two programs).

Figure 2.1: Comparison of Medicaid and Medicare Policy 1965-1983

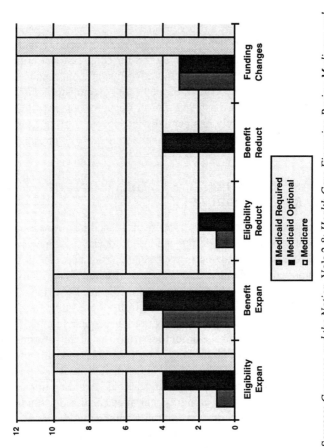

Sources: *Congress and the Nation*, Vols 2-8; *Health Care Financing Review Medicare and Medicaid Statistical Supplement, 1995; Social Security Bulletin, Annual Statistical Supplement, 1993.*

Methodology

In order to contrast the congressional treatment of medicaid and medicare, their legislative histories were examined in depth. Provisions dealing directly with *recipients* and the *financing* of the two programs were the primary focus of this investigation. Given the number and complexity of amendments to Titles XVIII (medicare) and XIX (medicaid) between 1966 and 1983, and because the selection of provisions required a judgment about the importance of certain provisions, and not merely a count of their number, a strategy was employed that assisted in the selection of the most substantial and relevant measures. Those measures included in *Congress and the Nation (C&N)* were deemed to be the major changes in the medicaid and medicare programs since 1965. However, because of the great number of changes included in most social security amendments, even the editors of that journal occasionally failed to include a measure which later proved significant (e.g., The Early and Periodic Screening, Diagnosis, and Treatment Program adopted in 1967 was not highlighted by *C&N* that year.) Consequently, *C&N*'s list was supplemented with other references, principally the *Social Security Bulletin, Annual Statistical Supplement, 1992*. In addition, other secondary sources (Rosenbaum 1993b; Stevens and Stevens 1974; and Thompson 1981) assisted in identifying important medicaid provisions that altered benefits, eligibility, or funding not featured in the above works.

In this way, a concise picture of the character of congressional treatment of beneficiaries and of changes in medicaid and medicare funding was shaped. A summary of the expansions and reductions in eligibility and benefits, as well as changes in funding for both programs, has been outlined in tables. Also, in order to give the reader a better sense of the trends in congressional treatment, these have been analyzed numerically as well. This numerical analysis must be interpreted with caution, however, because this analysis make no attempt to measure the scope or significance of the changes. Furthermore, related provisions in the same legislation and have often been lumped together and counted as one expansion or reduction in benefits.[4] Consequently, the numbers and graphs are designed to provide a sense of the frequency of the various types of congressional changes in the programs, rather than their breadth.

Expansions in Eligibility

Although Congress chose to expand eligibility for both programs, the scope of the expansions differed. While Congress adopted two very costly expansions in medicare eligibility during this period, it adopted one minor mandatory extension in medicaid eligibility.[5] Rather than requiring states to expand medicaid, when Congress chose to liberalize that program's eligibility, it allowed the states to determine whether to participate or not. (See Table 2.1 for a comparison of medicare and medicaid expansions in eligibility.)

The first optional expansion in medicaid eligibility occurred in 1972 when Congress nationalized eligibility for Supplemental Security Income. This also nationalized medicaid eligibility for the poor blind, elderly, and disabled. However, because of strong opposition by some states, Congress permitted them to retain more restrictive standards for determining medicaid eligibility if they chose (*Medicaid Source Book* 1993, 201-205).[6] Congress did not again extend eligibility for medicaid until the early 1980s. In 1981 and 1982 it permitted states to extend eligibility to disabled children cared for at home who would otherwise only be eligible if they were institutionalized. Congress also allowed states for the first time to consider poor, pregnant women an independent category of medicaid eligible in 1981. Prior to that time, a poor pregnant woman without children, who otherwise met the income and resource qualifications, might become eligible for medicaid only after she delivered her child. This measure would allow prenatal care for first-time mothers to be covered in an attempt to prevent low birth weights and forestall their accompanying exorbitant health care expenses.

Although Congress did not enact mandatory expansions in medicaid eligibility during this period, it did adopt five provisions protecting the eligibility of poor elderly and disabled medicaid recipients at risk of losing it due to changes in other related laws. It showed little comparable consideration for the eligibility of AFDC-related recipients.

In contrast to these relatively minor adjustments in medicaid eligibility, Congress extended medicare to two sizable and expensive groups. In 1972 eligibility was expanded to include those persons who were disabled for more than two years and to those suffering from end-

Table 2.1: Comparison of Expansions in Eligibility for Medicaid and Medicare: 1965-1983

| Year | Medicaid | | Medicare |
	Required	Optional	
1966			1 extended deadline for enrolling in **part B**
1972	• maintained eligibility for 4 months for recipients who would otherwise lose it due to 20% hike in OASDI benefits [1] • extended retroactive eligibility for 3 months for those found eligible (including the deceased)	• nationalized eligibility for welfare for the aged, blind, and disabled, but section 209 (b) of this provision permitted states to continue using their previous standards for determining medicaid eligibility	• extended eligibility to include 1.7 million disabled less than 65 years of age • extended eligibility to include individuals with End Stage Renal Disease (ESRD) • extended eligibility in **Part A** to those over 65 years who are enrolled in **Part B** but are not otherwise entitled to **Part A** benefits, to pay a monthly premium to participate in **Part A** • expanded **Part B** eligibility to those less than 65 years old entitled to **Part A** who pay the premium

Table 2.1 (continued)

| Year | Medicaid | | Medicare |
	Required	Optional	
1973	• maintained eligililily for 125,000 *essential persons* (spouses of SSI recipients who would otherwise lose it under SSI regulations)[1] • extended protection for 9 months for medicaid recipients from losing eligibility due to 1972 hike in OASDI benefits[1]		
1976	• Preserves medicaid eligibility of recipients who become ineligible for cash SSI payments due to changes in the COLA in OASDI benefits[1] • Protected married SSI recipients from a loss of medicaid benefits while the spouse was hospitalized[1]		

Table 2.1 (continued)

Year	Medicaid Required	Medicaid Optional	Medicare
1980			• extended eligibility to disabled who lost coverage due to employment • eliminated second waiting period for disabled if entitled again within 5 years • repealed limits on re-enrollment in **part B**
1981		• allowed waivers for home-and community-based care (only for those who would otherwise be cared for in an institution)	
1982		• extended eligibility to pregnant women who would otherwise be eligible after the birth of her child • expanded eligibility to home care for disabled children who would otherwise only be eligible as institutional recipients of SSI	• made certain federal employees eligible and required them to pay HI tax, despite the fact that 80% were already eligible
1983			• required all employees of non-profit organizations to join medicare and pay HI tax

1. These measures were not actually expansions, but protections for certain beneficiaries from cutbacks due to other policy changes.
Sources: *Congress and the Nation*, Vols. 2-6; *Health Care Financing Review Medicare and Medicaid Statistical Supplement*, 1992; *Annual Statistical Supplement to the Social Security Bulletin*, 1993.

stage renal disease. This legislation added 900,000 new enrollees and $1 billion to medicare expenditures by 1975; and by 1980 those figures had swollen to more than 1.5 million new enrollees and $2.8 billion (Social Security Administration 1993, 75, 310). The projection of low costs for these additional groups aided passage of these expansions; however, as with medicaid, the actual expenditures were grossly underestimated. Despite the large fiscal impact of these changes, Congress further eased eligibility for the disabled in 1980, permitting those who lost coverage due to employment to continue receiving benefits. In addition, Congress enlarged the number of those eligible for medicare in 1982 and again in 1983 by requiring certain federal employees and all employees of non-profit organizations to pay the Hospital Insurance premiums, thus enabling them to qualify for medicare benefits upon reaching age 65.

Expansions in Benefits

Although Congress adopted numerous enlargements in medicare benefits, it was reluctant to require the states to expand medicaid benefits. (See Table 2.2 for a comparison of medicare and medicaid expansions in benefits.) Among the many expansions for the medicare program were extensions in the duration and types of inpatient and outpatient services covered, including rural clinic services, home health visits, mental health services, and hospice care.

Medicaid's expansions were not as extensive, and were largely limited the first seven years of the program. When expanding medicaid benefits, Congress preferred to grant states an option. The first and most controversial expansion occurred very shortly after the creation of medicaid. In 1967 Congress created the Early Periodic, Screening, Diagnosis and Treatment Program (EPSDT). This was a very expensive and burdensome program for the states, requiring them to seek out all eligible poor children in need of care and to extend specialized services to them. This program instructed states to assess:

> their physical or mental defects, and provide such health care,
> treatment, and other measures to correct or ameliorate defects and
> chronic conditions discovered thereby, as may be provided for in
> regulations by the Secretary (Social Security Amendments of 1967,
> Sec. 1905 a 4 B).

Table 2.2: Comparison of Major Expansions in Benefits for Medicaid and Medicare: 1965-1983

Year	Medicaid		Medicare
	Required	**Optional**	
1967	• established Early and Periodic Diagnosis, Screening and Treatment program (EPSDT)	• allowed states to purchase part B medicare for *medically needy* elderly (not just welfare recipients) • allowed states to add coverage for welfare beneficiaries in intermediate care facilities (ICFs)	• added 60 days "lifetime reserve" for in-patient services • added ancillary hospital services and extended care facility services • added out-patient physical therapy and diagnostic x-rays, and purchase of durable medical equipment
1971		• permitted states to cover services for the *medically needy* provided in ICFs and ICFs for the mentally retarded	
1972	• added family planning services	• permits states to cover care for beneficiaries under 22 years old in psychiatric facilities (1965 legislation included care for those under 65 years) • extended coverage of optometrists and chiropractors	• added services of residents of podiatry training, outpatient physical therapy, chiropractic, speech pathology, and some optometry services.
1977	• added new health practitioners in rural clinics		• added new health practitioners in rural clinics

Table 2.2 (continued)

| Year | Medicaid | | Medicare |
	Required	Optional	
1980	• added nurse-midwife services		• removed limits on home health visits • authorized payments without the usual cost-sharing requirement for outpatient alcohol treatment, diagnostic tests, and certain surgical procedures • increased ceiling on outpatient physical therapy • extended coverage for outpatient services
1982			• added hospice services

Sources: *Congress and the Nation, Vols 2–6; Annual Statistical Supplement to the Social Security Bulletin,* 1993.

The ambiguous language of this statute and the intrusive regulations tentatively issued by the MSA created serious opposition within the states. Because of this, the Senate Finance Committee proposed an amendment to the Social Security Amendments of 1970 to scale back the requirements. Although that legislation was side-tracked, Congress gave clear signals to MSA that the regulations were to be narrower in scope (Stevens and Stevens 1974, 246-248). The states continued to resist implementation of this program, and eventually Congress withdrew even its symbolic efforts to support enforcement of these regulations. In 1981 it repealed the 1 percent penalty for noncompliance, which had never actually been imposed.

Besides enlarging the pool of medicaid providers to include practitioners in rural clinics and nurse midwives, Congress passed only one other minor required extension in medicaid services. In 1972, it added family planning to the list of services states were required to offer.

Rising Expenditures

Almost immediately after the implementation of the two programs, their costs exceeded all expectations. (See Table 2.3 for the rate of growth in expenditures for the two programs.) Based upon data from the first few years, a 1970 Report from the Staff of the Committee on Finance explained,

> The Department of Health, Education, and Welfare had estimated at the time Congress was considering the legislation that the Medicaid program would cost the Federal Government an additional $238 million in its first full year of operation. In fact, the Federal share of vendor payments for calendar year 1966 was precisely $238 million more than in calendar 1965—but only six States had programs in operation during the full year.
>
> In January 1967, the President's budget predicted that 48 States would have medicaid programs in operation by July 1, 1968, and that total payments would be $2.25 billion in fiscal year 1968 . . . Actual expenditures, with 37 States having medicaid programs, were $3.53 billion (Senate Finance Committee, hereafter SFC, Print 1970, 42).

Likewise costs of medicare's growth were underestimated. The same report states:

> In 1965 when medicare was enacted, the insurance program for payment of hospital bills was estimated to cost 1.23 percent of taxable payroll [based upon $6,600 of individual annual wages] . . . After only three years of experience, the conservative assumptions have been abandoned due to soaring costs resulting from price increases and greater-than-anticipated utilization of covered services. . . . Boiled down to dollars . . . the estimated cost for calendar year 1970 has jumped from the original projection of $3.1 billion to a current estimate of $5.8 billion (3).

Table 2.3: Medicaid and Medicare Expenditures: 1966-1983 ($ in millions)

Year	Medicaid			Medicare
	Federal	State/Local	Total	
1966	$ 635	$ 676	$3311	$ 1,728
1967	1,532	1,624	3,156	5,054
1968	1,843	1,715	3,558	6,164
1969	2,309	1,886	4,195	7,116
1970	2,856	2,459	5,315	7,633
1971	3,828	2,900	6,728	8,495
1972	4,568	3,783	8,351	9,299
1973	4,954	4,509	9,463	10,745
1974	6,301	4,815	11,116	13,458
1975	7,437	6,060	13,497	16,402
1976	9,165	6,093	15,258	19,790
1977	9,969	7,551	17,520	22,832
1978	10,940	8,594	19,534	26,780
1979	12,755	9,649	22,404	31,079
1980	14,499	11,635	26,134	37,533
1981	17,220	13,150	30,370	45,152
1982	17,487	14,644	32,131	52,642
1983	19,233	16,082	35,315	59,906

Source: U.S. House. 1993. Committee on Energy and Commerce. Subcommittee on Health and the Environment. *Medicaid Source Book.* 1993, 109.

Between 1966 and 1967, medicaid expenditures had more than doubled from $1.3 to $3.2 billion.[7] From 1965 to 1970, medicare expenditures grew even more rapidly—at an average annual rate of 45 percent, compared with medicaid's 41.9 percent. During the next five years, medicaid's yearly rate of growth outpaced that of medicare, averaging 20.5 percent versus medicare's 16.5 percent (*Medicaid Source Book* 1993, 109). Much of this expenditure increase can be explained by the rapid rise in the number of medicaid beneficiaries. From 1968 to 1978 the number of recipients doubled—increasing from 11 to 22 million (*Medicaid Source Book* 1993, 88-89). By comparison, medicare enrollees grew from 19.5 million in 1967 to 22.8 million in 1975 (DHHS 1993, 304).

Cost Control: Targeting Providers

In response, Congress initiated a variety of mild regulatory strategies to promote efficiency among health care providers. One of the early approaches, enacted in 1972, was to establish Professional Standard Review Organizations charged with monitoring the need and quality of care to patients financed by medicaid and medicare. Funds were also allocated for the development of Health Maintenance Organizations in 1973 in hopes of creating competition with the predominant, inflationary, fee-for-service system. In 1975 Congress passed the National Health Planning and Resource Development Act, which set up the national designation of local health systems areas designed to diminish the rapid growth and unnecessary duplication of medical facilities throughout the nation.[8] In 1967, 1968, and again in 1980, Congress imposed requirements on states to monitor utilization and improve nursing home services. Furthermore, Congress instituted measures to detect and correct fraud and abuse in both programs in the late 1970s and early 1980s.

As these attempts proved ineffective in controlling costs, Congress enacted even more intrusive interventions (Brown 1983). Despite the objections of health care providers, Congress finally tackled the inflationary cost-based method of reimbursement used in both programs. Through the Boren Amendments of 1980 and 1981, Congress granted states the freedom to adopt more efficient and innovative medicaid payment schemes for nursing homes and hospitals.[9] Then, in 1983, in the face of rapidly escalating costs and impending insolvency in medicare's Hospital Insurance trust fund, Congress undertook a new prospective approach to paying medicare providers.[10] These measures reveal Congress's willingness to target health care providers in its attempt to curtail medicare expenditures.

Cost-Control: Targeting of Beneficiaries

As the cost-spiral persisted, Congress undertook several other approaches to address it. What is most interesting, however, is how its strategies for dealing with the same problem—rising costs—differed for the medicaid and medicare programs. During this period, Congress enacted no curtailments in benefits or eligibility for the medicare program.[11] Instead, it energetically sought politically acceptable ways to expand its financing. But it did not do the same for medicaid. Congress sought to reduce that program's expenditures by curtailing funding to the states, cutting back eligibility and benefits, and granting states greater discretion to limit the scope of their programs. (See Table 2.4 for a comparison of the difference in the reductions of benefits and eligibility and Table 2.5 for changes in funding.)

One of the congressional strategies to slow the growth of federal medicaid expenditures was to reduce the scope of the program. As early as August 1966, the House Ways and Means Committee began closed-door hearings to discuss plans to control medicaid expenditures. The report issued from those hearings proposed a reduction in federal reimbursement for some of the most politically vulnerable groups (Stevens and Stevens 1974, 116). Although that recommendation was not adopted, other reductions in medicaid eligibility soon followed.

In 1967, Congress decided to limit eligibility for the *medically needy*. The original medicaid statutes placed no ceiling on eligibility for this category of medicaid beneficiaries. (See footnote 2 of this chapter for more thorough discussion of the various categories of medicaid eligibility.) Because of the incentives inherent in the medicaid matching funds, several states sought to exploit this category of eligibility as a means of substituting federal funds for their own. New York, for example, which had a generous state-financed health care program, made eligibility for the *medically needy* so generous that 45 percent of the population would have been eligible for medicaid (Stevens and Stevens 1974, 92). Fearful that states would raid the federal treasury to

Table 2.4: Comparison of Medicaid and Medicare Reductions in Eligibility and Benefits: 1965-1983

Year	Medicaid		Medicare
	Required	Optional	
1969		• allowed states to delay beginning steps towards comprehensiveness until 7/1/71 and extended deadline for requiring states to establish comprehensive coverage from 1975 to 1977 • permitted states to curtail *nonbasic* services[1]	• none
1972		• repealed 1902 (d) provision established in 1965 that required establishment of comprehensive medicaid coverage and maintenance of effort within states	• none
1980		• permitted states to restrict eligibility of those aged 18 to 21 under AFDC program to those in high school or vocational educational programs	• none

Table 2.4 (continued)

Year	Medicaid		Medicare
	Required	Optional	
1981	• tightened eligibility for AFDC, eliminating the inclusion of unborn children and 440,000 working poor families	• gave states with *medically needy* programs greater authority to limit coverage • allowed states to end medicaid coverage when a youth reached 19 rather than 21 years of age	• none

1. Congress also required states desiring to curtail services to prove they were applying cost-control measures to medicaid administration and not increasing reimbursement to providers

Sources: *Congress and the Nation, Vols 2-6; Annual Statistical Supplement to the Social Security Bulletin, 1993.*

Table 2.5: Comparison of Medicaid and Medicare Changes in Funding: 1965-1983

| Year | Medicaid | | Medicare |
	Required	Optional	
1967	• established that the federal government would only provide matching funds to states where medicaid eligibility permitted the *medically needy* to earn no more than 150% of the state income standard for the ADFC assistance program. This limit would decrease to 133% in 1970.		• allowed states to purchase **Part B** medicare for the *medically needy* (not just for welfare recipients) •increased the taxable wage base for **Part A** from $6,600 to $7,800 and phased in and increase in the contribution rate beginning 1/68 to a total of 5.9% (OASDI and HI) in 1987
1972			• limited the premium rate that beneficiaries paid for medicare **Part B** to the rate of increase in Old Age, Survivors, and Disability Insurance (OASDI) cash benefits • increased cost of deductible by $10 for **Part B** services

Table 2.5 (continued)

| Year | Medicaid | | Medicare |
	Required	Optional	
1972 (cont.)			• phased in an increase in the OASDHI tax rate and taxable income to to 5.85 % and $12,600 in 1974 over previous law (This represented a .4% increase in HI tax)
1973			• increased Social Security payroll tax wage base to $13,200 from $12,600 beginning 1/1/74 • altered tax rates among Social Security trust funds, increasing OASDI by 0.1% while decreasing HI by 0.1%
1981	• reduced federal matching rates for 3 years for states whose payments exceeded certain targets: reductions of 3% in fiscal 1982, 4% in 1983, and 4.5% in 1984.		• moderately increased the deductible for **Part A** and **Part B** services • eliminated carryover of incurred expenses from previous year for meeting **Part B** deductible

Table 2.5 (continued)

Year	Medicaid		Medicare
	Required	**Optional**	
1982	• reduced federal payment to states whose error rates exceed new federal standards	• permitted states to impose liens on home of institutionalized persons under certain circumstances	• expanded HI tax base by making certain federal employees eligible for medicare, requiring them to pay HI tax • increased the share the elderly would otherwise pay for **Part B** by setting the premium costs at one-fourth the cost of the program for elderly beneficiaries
1983			• expanded tax base by making employees of non-profit organizations eligible for medicare, requiring them to pay HI tax

Sources: *Congress and the Nation, Vols 2-6; Annual Statistical Supplement to the Social Security Bulletin, 1993.*

provide health care financing to a large population of the near-poor, Congress decided to limit the number of *medically needy* by linking eligibility for medicaid to income levels for cash assistance in each state. Beginning in 1967, states would receive no matching funds for the *medically needy* whose income exceeded 150 percent of that permitted for AFDC eligibility.[12]

Another important example of how Congress attempted to reduce the size of the medicaid program occurred early in that program's history. Although the original statutes were vague about the ultimate goal of the medicaid program, they were clear that states were expected to enlarge their programs. It mandated that they move "in the direction of broadening the scope of care and services available," and "in the direction of liberalizing the eligibility requirements for medical service" (Social Security Amendments 1965, Section 1903). However, Congress began compromising this requirement as early as 1969 when it extended the deadline for requiring states to establish comprehensive coverage, allowed them to delay even beginning to take steps toward comprehensiveness until 1971, and permitted them to curtail *non-basic* services.[13] The retreat from the goal of comprehensiveness was completed in 1972 when Congress repealed the initial provision. This action opened the door for states to institute a number of cutbacks. And so they did. In response to the relaxation of federal requirements in 1972, states initiated numerous cost controls, including "benefit limitations, requirements for prior authorization of services, and reductions in payment levels" (*Medicaid Source Book*, 1993, 31).

Then, again in the early 1980s, as fiscal pressures assumed prominence on the congressional agenda, instead of expanding the funding base for medicaid as it had done for medicare, Congress responded by curtailing that program. In 1981 Congress enacted its most direct assault on medicaid eligibility to date. The Omnibus Budget Reconciliation Act (OBRA) enacted that year tightened eligibility requirements for AFDC, eliminating approximately 442,000 working poor families from medicaid enrollment (Oberg and Polich 1988, 85). Through that same legislation, Congress also took the drastic step of reducing the federal matching rate for medicaid for three years by 3, 4 and 4.5 percent. Furthermore, it gave states greater freedom to curtail their medicaid programs by allowing them to end coverage to youths between the ages of 18 and 21 previously covered by AFDC, and to limit coverage for the *medically needy*.

In response to these congressional measures, many states cut services and reimbursement and limited eligibility (*Medicaid Source Book* 1993, 35). These programmatic changes, along with a drop of inflation during this period, helped to reduce the average annual growth rate for medicaid from 17 percent between 1979 and 1981 to 7 percent from 1982 to 1984.[14]

In contrast, medicare growth outpaced that of all other federal health care expenditures between 1972 and the mid-1980s (*Medicaid Source Book* 1993, 107-109). Instead of cutting back that program between 1965 and 1983, Congress initiated a number of measures to expand its financing. These will be discussed below.

RATIONALE FOR DIFFERING LEVELS OF SUPPORT

The puzzle posed by the Medicare/Medicaid comparison is why the two programs, simultaneously launched, should have produced such similar results medically and economically but had such different political fates. Both programs redistributed access in the intended direction (toward the old and the poor, respectively), both contributed substantially to medical inflation, and both put considerable pressure on government budgets at the federal and state levels. Why should Medicaid be regarded as a political scandal and subject to programmatic instability and Medicare remain so stable and, broadly speaking, legitimate? (Marmor 1983, xv)

Marmor offers a solution to the puzzle. He writes, "The answer lies in the political constituencies affected and the ideological claims they excited" (1983, xv). These two factors help to explain the difference in congressional treatment of medicaid and medicare between 1965 and 1983.

Ideology

Medicare and medicaid are grounded in different ideologies. One is quite strong and stable; while the other is more susceptible to change in public acceptance. These different ideologies have exerted great influence in shaping their different politics. Skocpol contrasts the two:

... Americans make a sharp conceptual and evaluative distinction between "social security" and "welfare." *Social Security* refers to old-age insurance and the associated programs of survivors, disability, and medical coverage for the elderly; and these programs are seen as sacred governmental obligations to deserving workers who have paid for them through "contributions" over their working lifetimes. *Welfare*, by contrast, is often discussed as a set of governmental "handouts" to barely deserving poor people who may be trying to avoid honest employment—trying to get something for nothing (1988, 296).

Medicare is a form of social insurance that has near universal coverage among the elderly; it is based upon the concept of individualism and self-sufficiency. These are deeply held American values that have remained stable over time. Thus, for medicare, the strength and constancy of these values have complemented its broad and stable distributional support. Ideological support for medicaid, on the other hand, rests largely upon the commitment to public assistance for the needy. The decision of Congress in 1965 to separate these two programs and to assign medicaid to a welfare administrative home, and medicare to the popular Social Security administration reveals the weaker level of support for medicaid. It also served to cement their separate ideological identities.

The ability of medicaid advocates to build support for their program has been hampered by the ongoing question regarding the "worthiness" of its recipients. An attempt to limit medicaid to the worthy poor has produced a complex and narrow set of eligibility categories, including those eligible by virtue of SSI, the poor elderly, blind, and disabled, and those eligible by virtue of AFDC, poor children and their single mothers.[15] Differences in the worthiness of these groups helps explain why during this period Congress has consistently treated SSI recipients with greater care than those associated with AFDC.

Since the 1960s, the number of AFDC recipients has mushroomed. Patterson indicates that "the number of Americans on public assistance grew from 7.1 million in 1960 ... to 14.4 million in 1974, and all of this growth came in the numbers on AFDC, which increased from 3.1 million in 1960 ... to 10.8 million in 1974" (1981, 171). The perception that AFDC recipients are morally deserving, never very strong, has fallen precipitously over the past two decades, both because of the rise in single-mothers on its rolls and the influence of race. The rate of unwed mothers, an increasing proportion of medicaid recipients, is on the rise, and this phenomenon is seen disproportionately among blacks.[16] Thus, due to the influence of race and questions about morality, the perception that a large segment of medicaid recipients are unworthy has contributed to weaker ideological support for this program.

Slessarev points out the demographic differences in the composition of medicare and medicaid, which further weakens the strength of medicaid's support. Although many elderly qualify for both programs, she shows how greatly the overall composition of the two programs differs. Medicare beneficiaries are overwhelmingly white, elderly, and non-poor; only 12.5 percent are minorities. Medicaid recipients are, on the other hand, poor and disproportionately non-white; over one-third are minorities (1988, 358).

Because medicaid's ideological appeal has been weaker, congressional support for that program has also been weaker. As federal expenditures began to exceed expectations, conservatives in Congress, especially Senator Long (D-LA), Chair of the Senate Finance Committee in the late 1960s, sought to diminish the scope of and federal commitment to the program. In 1968, for example, Long reintroduced an amendment to curtail the federal contribution to medicaid from the 50 to 83 percent range down to the 25 to 69 percent range.[17]

Ferejohn explains how support for welfare programs such as medicaid are influenced by elections. He writes,

> while the distributional features tend to remain stable over time . . . the ideological composition of Congress may fluctuate significantly over relatively short periods . . . Thus, programs based on ideological support are vulnerable to electorally induced shifts in the composition of Congress and in the executive (1991, 128).

Because of the different ideological bases of the two programs, medicaid's reliance upon liberal values in Congress left it more vulnerable in 1981 when a very conservative Congress took office. In that year, medicaid experienced the most serious mandatory reductions in federal funding and eligibility since its creation.

Distribution of Benefits

In addition to ideology, the distribution of policy benefits to important political constituencies is an important factor in determining the political support of all social welfare programs. Ferejohn employs this variable to help explain the behavior of individual members of Congress, of congressional committees, and ultimately of Congress as a whole concerning social welfare programs. He argues that both medicaid and medicare depend upon the broad distribution of their benefits as the major source of their political support (1991). Using this logic, when comparing the two programs, medicare has the advantage because its primary constituents—the elderly—are well-organized, widely distributed across all congressional districts, and vote in great numbers. This provides members of Congress with incentives to be quite responsive to their interests.

The actual recipients of medicare are merely the most obvious beneficiaries; other groups benefit significantly, as well. Economist Paul Feldstein points out two important secondary medicare beneficiaries—families and health care providers (1988, 226). One of the architects of medicare, Robert Ball, explains how important appealing to the sons and daughters of the elderly was in helping to promote the passage of medicare in 1965. He claims that one of the most "effective" brochures was entitled, *Medicare for Three Generations* (1995, 67). This broad voting constituency helps to explain the congressional incentive to continually expand benefits and to avoid curtailing them at all costs.

By contrast, medicaid constituents—primarily the poor—tend to vote less consistently, are less well-mobilized, display weak commitment in supporting programs and are not as evenly distributed across congressional districts. Consequently, members of Congress have less incentive to expand benefits and protect recipients of this program. One important exception involves a relatively small but significant population of medicaid recipients, those eligible by virtue of SSI—the poor elderly and disabled. Medicaid delivers important assistance to this group and their families.[18] This portion of the medicaid constituency, which overlaps with that of medicare, has enjoyed much stronger political support in Congress than the AFDC-related population.

Like the medicare program, medicaid also furnishes benefits to other, less obvious groups. Among the most influential have been health care providers who serve the poor. In 1981, for example, the support of hospitals helped to ward off even more damaging cut backs in the medicaid program. Slessarev explains,

> In Illinois almost half of all Medicaid payments go to hospitals, nearly $400 million in fiscal year 1982. This makes the program an important source of revenue for hospitals . . . That medicaid funding plays a crucial role in keeping many hospitals from closing was an argument made again and again by hospital administrators who testified in opposition to Reagan's proposed cap on Medicaid . . . Medicaid was saved from the Reagan ax by an exceptionally strong coalition of support that came to its rescue. The coalition consisted of neither Medicaid recipients or the AMA (1988, 374-376).

She points out another vitally important, but weaker, medicaid beneficiary, the states. Slessarev explains,

> . . . states have also become very dependent upon medicaid financing to assist with the cost of health care for the poor. . . . Medicaid came to have strong support among states and local politicians . . . In many states Medicaid is the largest program in the state's entire budget, while it is the predominant item in *every* state's health care budget. Therefore, cuts in the amount of federal funding for Medicaid would have serious repercussions for the states' budgets (1988, 375).

This issue was so important to governors that even Republican ones lobbied Reagan to spare medicaid in 1981 (Slessarev 1988, 375).

When threatened with losing an important federal grant, the states revealed their loyalty to certain aspects of medicaid. However, state policymakers display a mixed reaction to that program. Those features that promote the state's ability to shift part of the cost of care for the poor to the federal government are viewed as a blessing. But, those that impose unwanted regulations and costs upon them are a curse. Frank Thompson summarizes the states' view as follows,

> In general, lobbies for state officials supported medicaid measures that promised to save them money. They advocated in this respect . . .

increased federal subsidy of state administrative costs; greater
flexibility to implement alternative methods of paying providers;
federal assumption of all copayments and deductibles for Medicare
recipients . . . (1981, 119).

This difference in the breadth and scope of political influence of
the constituencies for these two programs and their different ideological
bases helps to explain the different levels of support for the two
programs. However, they only partially explain how Congress managed
to minimize opposition to medicare's rapidly rising costs, in contrast to
medicaid, and why Congress chose to cut back the medicaid program
while avoiding that option for medicare.

Distribution of Costs

Another important factor that helped produce different levels of support
for medicaid and medicare between 1965 and 1983 is the distribution of
costs associated with the programs. Whereas virtually every
government program imposes costs as well as benefits, congressional
policymakers seek to disperse or hide those costs in order to enhance a
program's political appeal (Arnold 1990). Congress designed
medicare's funding to be more complex, confusing, and more widely
dispersed than medicaid's. Furthermore, as costs increased, between
1966 and 1983 it repeatedly intervened to protect medicare
beneficiaries and disperse the costs of that program even more widely.
The lack of visibility and the diffusion of the impact of rising medicare
expenditures minimized controversy over that program's rising
expenditures.

Medicaid's funding mechanism, on the other hand, permitted its
expenditures to be more visible and concentrated, thus promoting early
and vocal opposition from the states . Furthermore, Congress
exacerbated this situation by adopting measures between 1966 and
1983 that concentrated medicaid costs even more. (See Table 2.5 for a
comparison of changes in funding for the two programs between 1966
and 1983.) Vocal opposition to medicaid's expenses from the states
helps to explain why Congress repeatedly granted the states increased
freedom to curtail their programs throughout the period.

Costs for medicare are spread over two parts, and funding for each
differs. Part A, Hospital Insurance (HI), is financed through payroll

deductions of current workers. By setting its initial rate quite low, only 0.35 percent,[19] and by attaching it to the larger Social Security tax, it remained relatively invisible. Wildavsky writes:

> Medicare is shielded through its relationship with social security. Social Security, approximately four times greater and longer in existence, takes a much larger share of the pie. Individuals tend to identify the payroll tax as "the social security tax," and many are more or less unaware of the portion being taken to finance medicare (1992, 311-312).

Medicare Part B, Supplementary Medical Insurance (SMI), which is voluntary, was designed to be financed one-half through premiums deducted from Social Security payments to individuals and one-half through the federal treasury. The initial premium was merely $3 per month. In reality, the cost of SMI was funded by both current taxpayers and future ones, to the extent that medicare expenditures contributed to the federal deficit. However, the costs associated with medicare are not funded by these sources alone. Those medicare beneficiaries who found it necessary to use that program's benefits were also subject to cost-sharing expenses. Both Part A and Part B users were required to pay a deductible, initially a modest $40 and $50 respectively; and Part B users were also required to pay twenty percent of the health care provider's charges.

Thus, the expenses associated with the medicare program were designed to fall to a number of groups in a complex arrangement of financing: current workers (HI tax), the beneficiaries of medicare (premiums for SMI), users of medicare (deductible and co-payments for HI and SMI), and current and future federal taxpayers (one-half of SMI). This method of financing assured the elderly would not bear the full brunt of their health care expenditures and minimized organized opposition from taxpayers to growth in that program's expenses.

As medicare's expenditures grew, Congress responded in ways that minimized the threat of resistance from taxpayers and beneficiaries who had to foot the ever-growing bill. It employed three strategies to help make the costs more politically palatable: It protected the beneficiaries from the true cost of the program; it dispersed the costs of financing medicare even more widely; and when necessary, it increased the burden on the various groups associated with medicare in an

Table 2.6: Medicare cost sharing and premium sharing: 1965 to 1983

Year	Hospital Insurance		Supplementary Medical Insurance		
	Inpatient Hospital Deductible	Monthly Premium for voluntary participation	Annual Deductible	Coinsurance	Monthly Premium for enrollee (aged and disabled)
1966	$40		$50	20%	$3.00
1967	40		50	20	3.00
1968	40		50	20	4.00
1969	44		50	20	4.00
1970	52		50	20	5.30
1971	60		50	20	5.60
1972	68		50	20	5.80
1973	72	$33	60	20	6.30
1974	84	36	60	20	6.70
1975	92	40	60	20	6.70
1976	104	45	60	20	7.20
1977	124	54	60	20	7.70
1978	144	63	60	20	8.20
1979	160	69	60	20	8.70
1980	180	78	60	20	9.60
1981	204	89	60	20	11.00
1982	260	113	75	20	12.20
1983	304	113	75	20	12.20

Source: U.S. Department of Health and Human Services. 1993. *Annual Statistical Supplement, 1993 to the Social Security Bulletin*, 87.

incremental manner. Handling rapidly rising expenditures in this way helped to maintain support and minimize opposition to the program. (See Table 2.6 for the incremental increase in costs associated with medicare.)

Congress protected the beneficiaries of Part B from the rapid increase in expenditures by shifting costs to federal taxpayers. Although SMI premiums were initially designed to finance half the cost of this benefit, Congress intervened in 1972 to limit the increase that beneficiaries paid for SMI to the rate of increase in OASDI benefits. Because of this, the proportion of program costs financed by beneficiaries decreased from 47 percent in 1974 to 24 percent in 1982 (*C&N* Vol. 6, 535). Therefore, over time, beneficiaries paid smaller portions of part B expenditures than initially intended.

Congress also curbed opposition to rising expenditures by ensuring that costs would be dispersed as widely as possible. It did so by requiring new groups to pay the HI tax. An example of this strategy occurred in 1982 when Congress made certain federal employees eligible for medicare, and required them to pay the HI tax. This was not done as a beneficent gesture, but rather primarily as a means of increasing medicare revenues, since eighty percent of the retired federal employees at the time were eligible for medicare by virtue of their earlier private sector employment or their spouse's employment without paying the tax as federal employees (*C&N* Vol. 6, 534). Congress similarly made all employees of non-profit organizations eligible in 1983, requiring them also to pay the HI tax.

A third strategy to make higher taxes and beneficiary cost-sharing more acceptable was to ensure that they occurred incrementally. In order to keep the HI trust fund solvent, Congress instituted an automatic and gradual expansion in the HI tax rate and wage base to which current workers would be subject. However, because of unexpectedly rapid growth in expenditures, Congress intervened several times (1967, 1972, and 1973) to enlarge both the wage base and the tax rate beyond that set by previous law. (See Table 2.7 for the changes in taxable earnings and wage rate that occurred between 1966 and 1983.) Because of the close association of the HI tax with the highly regarded Social Security program these increases have gone largely unnoticed by the public. Wildavsky explains,

Between 1966 and 1982, the taxable wage base rose from $6,000 to $32,400, almost a fivefold increase. Over that same period the medicare tax rate increased from 0.7 to 2.6 percent. An individual with no change in income would have incurred a 270 percent increase in his medicare contribution over than period. And a person whose income matched or exceeded the wage base would have seen her annual contribution increase from $23.10 to $421.20, an increase of over 1,700 percent . . . (1992, 311-312).

Table 2.7: Annual Maximum Taxable Earnings and Contribution Rates for Old Age Survivors Insurance and Hospital Insurance: 1966-1983

Date	Annual maximum taxable earnings	Contribution Rate Employer/Employee Each	
		OASI	HI
1966	$6,600	3.5 %	0.35 %
1967	6,600	3.55	.5
1968	7,800	3.25	.6
1969	7,800	3.725	.6
1970	7,800	3.65	.6
1971	7,800	4.05	.6
1972	9,000	4.05	.6
1973	10,800	4.3	1.0
1974	13,200	4.375	.9
1975	14,100 [1]	4.375	.9
1976	15,300 [1]	4.375	.9
1977	16,500 [1]	4.375	.9
1978	17,700 [1]	4.275	1.0
1979	22,900	4.33	1.05
1980	25,900	4.52	1.05
1981	29,700	4.7	1.3
1982	32,400 [1]	4.575	1.3
1983	35,700 [1]	4.775	1.3

[1] Based on automatic adjustments under 1972 and 1973 statutes, increasing this amount in proportion to the increase in average wages.

Source: U.S. Department of Health and Human Services. 1993. *Annual Supplement, 1993 to the Social Security Bulletin,* 25.

It is remarkable that a tax increase of this magnitude produced hardly a ripple of opposition. Had Congress not expanded the wage base (but merely the tax rate) the costs would have been much more visible; and had these changes not been incremental, they would have been much more conspicuous, generating strong opposition.

By contrast, Congress did not disperse or hide medicaid expenditures nearly as successfully. That program was designed to derive its financing from the general revenues of the state and federal governments on a matching basis.[21] As with medicare's part B, the cost of the federal contribution to medicaid was dispersed among both current and future taxpayers. However, constitutional requirements in most states prohibited them from incurring a deficit; consequently, state medicaid expenditures were financed solely by current taxpayers in that state.[22] Furthermore, because of the nature of the clientele served by the medicaid program and statutory limitations, cost-sharing could not be imposed upon users of the program as it had been with medicare.[23]

This funding arrangement placed a heavy burden on state taxpayers. Because tremendous competitive pressure exists within each of the states to keep taxes low, especially for redistributive programs such as medicaid (Peterson, Rabe and Wong 1986), such an arrangement also placed state policymakers in a difficult position. They had to find politically acceptable means to finance this program. And their predicament worsened as medicaid's costs mushroomed.

A report issued by the Committee on Finance in 1970 revealed the extent of the burden medicaid placed upon the states from the very beginning. It says:

> Medical vendor payments have risen over the four year period from less than one-third to almost one-half of welfare expenditures (excluding the cost of administration). In absolute dollar terms, the rise has been precipitous: from $764 million in State and local funds . . . in fiscal year 1965 to an estimated $1,896 million in fiscal year 1968—a 150% increase within four years (SFC Print 1970, 44)

The states have always had a love-hate relationship with medicaid—they love the federal funds it brings them, but resent the heavy financial costs and administrative complexity of the program (Thompson 1981, 119). Nearly half the cost of medicaid falls to the states, which have relatively few options to deal with the rising expenditures associated with medicaid. They could reduce medicaid program expenses (through decreasing eligibility, benefits, or reimbursements to providers); increase taxes; curtail other state programs; or seek greater flexibility in the administration of the program from Congress. In fact, they pursued all of these options to varying extents. The staff of the Senate Finance Committee conducted a survey of governors in 1968 that revealed:

> One-third of the States initiating a medicaid program in 1966 or 1967 have raised taxes at least in part due to medicaid costs; a number of Governors states that the tax increases in their States could be directly linked to greater-than-anticipated medicaid costs. Several governors attributed either cutbacks in other State programs or curtailment of growth in other programs directly to increased medicaid costs (SFC Print 1970, 44).

The strain on state welfare budgets has "ensured increasing political unpopularity for medicaid, especially in terms of requiring additional taxes on those lower-income groups" according to Stevens and Stevens (1974, 160). As a result, significant opposition to the requirements of the medicaid program arose from the states. The Senate Finance Committee Report continues:

> One-third of the States that initiated medicaid programs in 1966 and 1967 have instituted or are planning to institute cutbacks in the scope or coverage of their medicaid programs as a result of cost-increases (SFC Print 1970, 44).

Because the inflexibility of the medicaid program imposed such visible and unwelcome costs upon the states, they appealed to Congress for relief of its requirements, especially in the early years of the program.

In response to state requests for greater flexibility, Congress complied in 1969 and 1972. States then curtailed their programs, but costs continued to grow. Medicaid absorbed one percent of state and local expenditures in 1966; by 1981 that had grown to 4.8 percent (*Medicaid Source Book* 1993, 114). By 1983 medicaid had grown to 5.1 percent of state and local expenditures (*Medicaid Source Book* 1993, 114). So again, in 1980, 1981, and 1982, in response to state pleas, Congress granted states further discretion over aspects of eligibility, benefits, and reimbursement of providers. (See Table 2.4 for optional reductions in eligibility and benefits.)

The funding arrangements for medicaid, which placed a heavy burden on state taxpayers, assured that as the costs of the program grew, opposition would too. Pressures on state policymakers to keep welfare expenditures low has meant that, from the very beginning, they would seek to curtail the mandatory aspects of the medicaid program. Because the costs of medicare were so much more widely dispersed, no comparable source of opposition emerged.

CONCLUSION

Medicaid did not enjoy the same level of congressional support as medicare between 1965 and 1983. The medicaid program suffered greater cutbacks, experienced fewer expansions, and its beneficiaries were not as well shielded from congressional cost-control efforts as those of medicare. Although differences in ideology and political constituencies help to explain this difference in treatment, the difference in funding for the two programs also played an important role in shaping their congressional politics.

Because medicaid had weaker and more variable ideological support and appealed to a less powerful constituency, that program did not enjoy the same consistent level of support as medicare. Furthermore, because medicaid's costs were not as widely dispersed as medicare's, when expenditures for both programs began to rise, significant opposition to medicaid emerged from within the states. No comparable organized opposition to medicare appeared.

NOTES

1. Thompson used this term to describe Congress's treatment of medicaid (1981, 121).

2. Eligibility for medicaid has always been very complex. The initial legislation laid out *four* different categories: Two were required: the *categorically needy-* those who received aid under the four categorically assistance programs (OAA, AB, AFDC, APTD); and the *categorically related needy-* those who would be included in these programs were it not for a specific state provision overridden by Title XIX (e.g., residence requirement). Two other categories of medicaid were optional: the *categorically related medically needy* and the *non-categorically related medically needy*. These categories

include those whose income exceeds limits set for cash assistance programs, but whose medical bills are so excessive as to bring their disposable income below the limit for cash assistance.

3. Congress did make several efforts to protect the small portion of medicaid recipients who were eligible by virtue of their eligibility for SSI.

4. For example, in 1972 Congress expanded the services of various types of health care providers to medicare recipients: residents of podiatry training, outpatient physical therapy, chiropractic, speech pathology, and optometry. I counted this as one expansion. However, in the same year, Congress added only family planning services to medicaid benefits. This expansion I also counted as one.

5. In 1972, for those who were determined to be eligible, it allowed a three month retroactive extension in eligibility.

6. Currently 12 states retain more restrictive eligibility standards.

7. This figure included expenditures for medicaid's predecessor Kerr-Mills, which was not phased out until December 31, 1969.

8. The National Health Planning and Resource Development Act created local health systems areas (HSAs), which contained representatives of health care providers, local governments, and consumers, and were charged with determining the need for new health care facilities within a particular area. They then made recommendations to state governments whether to permit such construction or not. The effectiveness of this approach in curtailing the growth of health care facilities has been marginal, at best. The recommendations of the HSA could be, and often were, ignored by state officials.

9. Although the Boren Amendments permitted states increased flexibility in establishing provider reimbursement systems, it also included some guidelines which only later grew in importance.

10. The amount a hospital would be paid by medicare would be determined in advance—based upon the beneficiary's age and diagnosis.

11. Congress did expand cost-sharing requirements for medicare beneficiaries during the early 1980s, which some analysts refer to as a *reduction in benefits,* but this is addressed under the topic of changes in funding.

12. This requirement became increasingly stringent, so that by 1970, when it was fully phased in, the income limit for medicaid became 133 percent of the ADFC income standard.

13. Congress required states desiring to curtail these *non-basic* services to prove they were applying cost-control measures to medicaid administration and not increasing reimbursement to providers.

14. When controlled for inflation, the annual rate of medicaid growth was -4.6 percent for 1982,-1.8 percent for 1983, and 1 percent in 1984 (*Medicaid Source Book* 1993, 96).

15. Eligibility for AFDC and SSI automatically assures eligibility for medicaid. In 1983, the number of medicaid beneficiaries eligible through AFDC equaled 15,127 million. The number eligible through SSI equaled 6,293 (*Medicaid Source Book* 1993, 160).

16. Between 1960 and 1983, the proportion of female-headed households with children increased from 6 to 14 percent among whites and from 21 to 48 percent among blacks, largely due to never having been married (Neckerman et al. 1988, 399).

17. Although this amendment passed the Senate, it ultimately failed to be adopted because of an outcry from the states and HEW (Stevens and Stevens 1974, 144).

18. Despite the fact that the elderly and disabled comprised only 29 percent of medicaid beneficiaries in 1981, over 70 percent of medicaid payments went to finance their care (*Medicaid Source Book* 1993, 160, 154).

19. The HI tax rate in 1966 was only 10 percent the size of the OASI tax rate.

20. The rate differs according to the per capita income of the state, with a minimum match of fifty percent.

21. States are also allowed to share the cost of medicaid with local governments, however, they must assure that 40 percent of the non-federal share comes from state sources. Few states actually have local governments help to finance medicaid. In 1991, only 14 states did (*Medicaid Source Book* 1993, 495).

22. Social Security Amendments of 1965, Section 1902 (a) (14) prohibited states from imposing cost-sharing on in-patient care and set guidelines for other sorts of cost-sharing. In 1972, Congress did permit some modest cost-sharing (co-payments and deductibles) for some of the medicaid recipients, but it was difficult for providers to collect these (Stevens and Stevens 1974, 339).Permission for states to require cost-sharing among medicaid recipients was expanded in 1982.

CHAPTER THREE

Congressional Treatment of Medicare and Medicaid: 1984 to 1990

Whereas during the first nineteen years of medicaid's existence Congress demonstrated lukewarm affection for the program, it developed an intense, if short-lived, love affair with it during the mid- and late-1980s. Congress chose to expand medicaid benefits and eligibility extensively and repeatedly between 1984 and 1990. At the same time, it proved unable to extend benefits for medicare recipients comparably. Instead, medicare costs were cut disproportionately. As a result of this surprising reversal in congressional behavior, the rate of growth in medicaid expenditures mushroomed while that for medicare leveled off. This chapter will contrast congressional treatment of the two programs during their earlier years with the years 1984 to 1990. (See Figure 3.1 for a summary of the comparisons.)

1984-1990 COMPARED WITH 1965-1983

Between 1984 and 1990 Congress enacted frequent medicaid expansions in sharp contrast to the previous 19 years. (See Table 3.1 for details of the expansions enacted from 1984 to 1990; and see Table 3.2 for a comparison of medicaid policy 1965-1983 with that of 1984-90.) Prior to 1984, Congress had adopted only one minor mandatory extension in eligibility, and four optional ones. However, during each of the seven years between 1984 and 1990, Congress chose to expand medicaid eligibility. Equally striking is the population targeted and the

Figure 3.1: Comparison of Number of Medicaid and Medicare Policy Changes: 1965-1983 and 1984-1990

1965- 1983

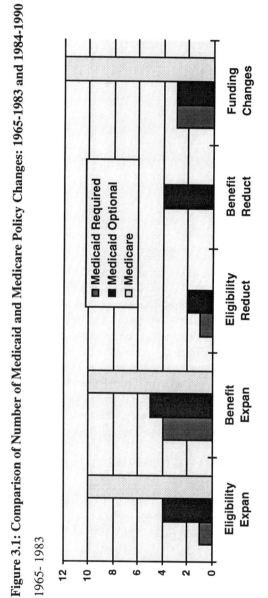

Figure 3.1 (continued)

1984 - 1990

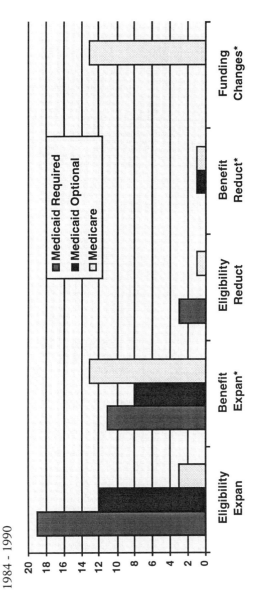

Sources: *Congress and the Nation*, Vols 2-8; *Social Security Bulletin, Annual Statistical Supplement*, 1993.

* The changes associated with the 1988 MCCA and its repeal are counted as one expansion, one repeal, and two changes in funding.

mandatory nature of the later expansions. During the earlier period, Congress went to great lengths to protect the SSI population, whereas after 1983, Congress demonstrated a remarkable change of preference. Although it still included the elderly among medicaid's new beneficiaries, Congress reserved its greatest demonstration of largess for poor and near-poor pregnant women, children and families. Furthermore, instead of permitting the states wide discretion regarding medicaid eligibility as it had historically done, Congress mandated 19 of the 31 extensions in eligibility that it adopted between 1984 and 1990.

It has always been relatively easy for Congress to increase benefits for medicaid. This may be because benefit increases usually are not as expensive as extensions in eligibility, and many of the advantages of expanding benefits accrue to health care providers as well as to recipients. Given the political incentives for doing so, it is not surprising that prior to 1984, Congress had already enacted four required and five optional expansions in benefits. Many of these were extensions in medicaid services to include various categories of health care providers, such as physical therapists, chiropractors, and speech pathologists. In 1985, 1986 and 1987 Congress enacted a total of 8 optional extensions in a wide range of benefits. But then it became even more determined. In the years 1988 through 1990, it adopted 9 more extensions in benefits—all mandatory. These measures extended coverage to new categories of providers and extended benefits to a variety of medicaid recipients. Again, Congress singled out pregnant women and children, not the elderly and disabled, for its most generous treatment. (See Table 3.3 for a summary of the extensions in benefits between 1984 and 1990.)

This stands in marked contrast to its behavior just a few years earlier. In 1982 and 1983, because of state and congressional cutbacks in eligibility, the number of children enrolled in AFDC (and medicaid) actually declined by 0.3 percent and 2.4 percent respectively, despite an increase in childhood poverty of 16 percent (*Medicaid Source Book* 1993, 35, 98-99; Holahan and Cohen 1986, 42-45). However, between 1987 and 1991, medicaid eligibility among children and adults (non-elderly and non-disabled) increased annually by 6.6 percent and 6 percent respectively. The number of enrollees in these categories increased from 12.1 to 16.5 million children and from 5.4 to 16.5

Table 3.1: Comparison of Expansions in Eligibility for Medicaid and Medicare: 1984-90

Year	Medicaid		Medicare
	Required	**Optional**	
1984	• mandated coverage of first-time pregnant women, pregnant women in two-parent families where the breadwinner was unemployed, and children (born after 10/1/83) up to age five in two-parent families	• permitted states to increase eligibility for AFDC and medicaid by raising the upper limit on family income from 150% to 185% of federal poverty level	
	• expanded eligibility for up to 15 months for employed persons losing AFDC due to changes in earned income disregards		
	• extended automatic eligibility to newborns of mothers receiving medicaid		
	• extended coverage for 4 months for children and caretakers who lose eligibility due to increased child support payments[1]		
	• raised assets SSI beneficiaries could have and still qualify		

Table 3.1 (continued)

| Year | Medicaid | | Medicare |
	Required	Optional	
1985	• extended medicaid coverage to pregnant women in two-parent, employed families who meet financial criteria for AFDC • extended medicaid for 60 days post-partum to women who received medicaid during pregnancy • restored medicaid to certain widows and widowers losing SSI and medicaid due to changes in OASDI actuarial methods[1]	• permitted states to extend medicaid to certain foster care and adoptive children	• extended eligibility to virtually all state and local employees hired after 12/31/85 for medicare **Part A** and required them to pay HI tax; made eligibility voluntary for those hired prior to that date • extended eligibility to all persons over 65 who pay a monthly premium
1986	• protected medicaid coverage for those enrolled in SSI that lose SSI due to earnings, who need medicaid to continue working, and whose earnings do not replace benefits lost	• permitted states to cover pregnant women, and children under age 5 (phased in) with family incomes below 100% of federal poverty level. Permits states to disregard assets.	

Table 3.1 (continued)

Year	Medicaid		Medicare
	Required	**Optional**	
1986 (cont.)		• allowed states to provide continuous coverage throughout pregnancy and post-partum regardless of changes in family income	
		• created new optional *categorically needy* group for aged and disabled with income below 100 percent of federal poverty line	
		• extended medicaid to otherwise eligible temporary resident aliens who are pregnant, children, or those with emergency medical conditions, elderly or disabled	

Table 3.1 (continued)

Year	Medicaid		Medicare
	Required	**Optional**	
1986 (cont.)		• allowed states that extended eligibility to pregnant women and children to use medicaid to pay for medicare cost-sharing expenses for qualified Medicare beneficiaries (QMB) with incomes up to 100 percent of the federal poverty level • clarified that state must make medicaid available to the homeless	
1987		• permitted states to cover all pregnant women and infants with incomes under 185% of the federal poverty level • allowed immediate expansion of OBRA 1986 coverage up to 100% of poverty line for children up to age 5 years	• permitted previously disabled individuals to resume coverage without 2 year wait

Table 3.1 (continued)

Year	Medicaid		Medicare
	Required	**Optional**	
1987 (cont.)		• allowed coverage for children aged 5-7, up to state AFDC levels (phased in) • allowed coverage for children below 9 years of age up to 100% of federal poverty level (phased in)	
1988	• made mandatory the OBRA 1986 option of providing medicaid coverage for pregnant women and infants with incomes up to 100% of the federal poverty level (phased) • made mandatory the OBRA 1986 option of states to pay for medicare cost-sharing expenses of QMBs with incomes up to 100% of the federal poverty level (phased in)	• permits states to establish more generous eligibility standards and methods for non-cash assistance medicaid applicants	

Table 3.1 (continued)

| Year | Medicaid | | Medicare |
	Required	Optional	
1988 (cont.)	• protected medicaid eligibility of AFDC recipients and the *medically needy* by prohibiting states from reducing AFDC payments below May 1988 levels93 increased required period of medicaid coverage if AFDC cash assistance is lost due to earnings[1]94 required medicaid coverage for two-parent unemployed families if otherwise eligible • liberalized rules for treatment of earned income for AFDC and medicaid purposes • protected medicaid eligibility of AFDC recipients and the *medically needy* by prohibiting states from reducing AFDC payments below May 1988 levels		

Table 3.1 (continued)

| Year | Medicaid | | Medicare |
	Required	Optional	
1989	• required states to extend coverage to pregnant women , infants, and children up to 6 years of age if income is below 133% of the federal poverty level		
1990	• required states to provide coverage to children up to age 18, if income is below 100% of the federal poverty level (phased in) • required states to provide coverage to women throughout the post-partum period that was made optional under OBRA 1986 • extended the period of presumptive eligibility for pregnant women before a written application was required		

Table 3.1 (continued)

Year	Medicaid		Medicare
	Required	**Optional**	
1990 (cont.)	• required states to receive and process applications for pregnant women and children at convenient outreach sites • required states to offer continuous eligibility to infants if they were born to a medicaid-eligible mother *and* remain in the mother's household • extended the MCCA *qualified Medicare beneficiary* provision to those with incomes below 120% of the federal poverty level (phased in)	• permitted certain states to liberalize *medically needy* income standard for a single person	

1. These measures were not actually expansions, but protections for certain beneficiaries from cutbacks due to other policy changes.
Sources: *Congress and the Nation*, Vols 6-8; *Social Security Bulletin, Annual Statistical Supplement, 1993*.

Table 3.2: Comparison of the Number of Medicaid Policy Changes: 1965-1983 and 1984-1990

Feature	1965-1983		1984-1990	
	Required	Optional	Required	Optional
Expansion in Eligibility	1	4	19	12
Expansion in Benefits	4	5	11	8
Reduction in Eligibility	1	2	3	none
Reduction in Benefits	none	4	none	1
Changes in Funding	3	3	none[1]	none

[1] Although there were no funding changes required of the states, Congress adopted four provisions that directed HCFA to protect the financial status of the states with regard to matching.funds.

Sources: *Congress and the Nation,* Vols 2-8; *Social Security Bulletin, Annual Statistical Supplement, 1993.*

Table 3.3: Comparison of Expansions in Benefits for Medicaid and Medicare: 1984-1990

| Year | Medicaid | | Medicare |
	Required	Optional	
1984			• extended outpatient services covered under **Part B**
1985		• permitted states to provide additional benefits to pregnant women not normally covered for other medicaid recipients • permitted states to cover habilitation services to those discharged from long term care settings who participate in home- and community-based programs • permitted states to cover home-and community based services whose costs exceed estimated institutional care • permitted states to cover hospice care	• expanded benefits to include liver transplants • made permanent coverage and increases reimbursement rates for hospice care

Table 3.3 (continued)

| Year | Medicaid | | Medicare |
	Required	Optional	
1985 (cont.)		• permitted states to extend case management services to some or all of their medicaid population	
1986		• permitted states to extend community-based care to those with AIDS and those with mental illness who would otherwise be institutionalized • permitted coverage of home care for the ventilator-dependent	• extended **Part A** and **B** coverage of certain services performed by non-physician providers, including occupational therapist, nurse anesthetists, optometrists • extended **Part B** surgical coverage to include those performed in outpatient settings
1987		• allowed home- and community-based services to the elderly who would otherwise need to be institutionalization • allowed states to pay the costs of health services delivered by clinics to the homeless	• increased coverage and reimbursement for mental health services • extended **Part B** coverage to non-physician providers, including: nurse-midwives, clinical psychologists, physician assistants

Table 3.3 (continued)

| Year | Medicaid | | Medicare |
	Required	Optional	
1988	• established higher minimum levels of protected income and assets for spouses of institutionalized individuals • clarifies state obligation to pay for education-related services to disabled children		• extended coverage to outpatient drugs and extended a number of other benefits to cover catastrophic medical expenses, limiting the financial risk to beneficiaries
1989	• required states to provide care needed to correct problems identified in children under the EPSDT program, even if not otherwise covered under state medicaid plan • required more frequent periodic screenings under the EPSDT program when medical problems are suspected		• expanded **Part B** coverage of non-physician health care providers in various settings • extended **Part B** coverage to include Pap smears • barred nursing homes from charging medicare patients more than the medicare-approved amount • eliminated **Part B** limits on mental health services

Table 3.3 (continued)

Year	Medicaid		Medicare
	Required	**Optional**	
1989 (cont.)	• required states to cover pediatric nurse practitioner services to the extent such services are permitted by state law • required that state reimbursement of medicaid providers be *sufficient* to ensure that services are as adequate for medicaid recipients as they would be for the general public • required states to include Federally Qualified Health Centers as medicaid providers and to reimburse them 100% of reasonable costs • required states to pay Part A premiums for certain qualified working disabled		

Table 3.3 (continued)

Year	Medicaid		Medicare
	Required	**Optional**	
1990	• required states to pay health insurance premiums where cost effective and pay other cost-sharing for beneficiaries who are otherwise eligible for private insurance • required states to receive and process applications for pregnant women and children at convenient outreach sites • required states to offer continuous eligibility to infants if they were born to a medicaid-eligible mother *and* remain in the mother's household		• extended length of hospice benefits beyond 210 days (had been in the 1988 MCCA which was repealed in 1989) • expanded coverage to include mammograms, injectable drugs for osteoporosis, Erythropoietin for ESRD

Sources: *Congress and the Nation*, Vols 6-8; *Social Security Bulletin, Annual Statistical Supplement, 1993.*

million adults between 1984 and 1991. Holahan et al. (1993) suggest that congressionally mandated expansions were a major reason. Extensions for pregnant women and children alone were responsible for increasing medicaid enrollment by 13.2 percent in 1990, and for approximately 22 percent of medicaid's expenditure growth between 1985 and 1990. Expenditures for children enrolled in medicaid grew from $4.4 billion in 1984 to $13.2 in 1991 (Holahan et al. 1993, 24, 29).

Reductions in Eligibility and Benefits

Taking benefits or eligibility away from some group that once possessed them is one of the most politically difficult tasks, because it arouses a protective response from the affected group and their allies (Arnold 1990). Nevertheless, because of fiscal pressure on both levels of government and the low political efficacy of medicaid recipients, Congress repeatedly granted the states greater freedom to reduce their medicaid benefits and eligibility between 1966 and 1983. In 1981 Congress directly assaulted the medicaid program, tightening eligibility for AFDC recipients and eliminating thousands of working poor from the medicaid rolls. After 1983, Congress changed its course. (See Table 3.2 for a comparison of earlier and later medicaid policy; and Table 3.4 for a list of the reductions in benefits and eligibility enacted between 1984 and 1990). It legislated only three required restrictions in eligibility, and two of these were reasonable attempts to prevent exploitation of the program by those who had other resources to pay for their health care. The third eliminated illegal aliens. Only one other reduction occurred during this period. It was optional, and allowed states to deny coverage for medically necessary, but often very expensive, non-experimental organ transplants.

Changes in Funding

Between 1965 and 1983, Congress reduced its commitment to fund medicaid and increased the burden upon states for financing medicaid expenditures.[1] Between 1984 and 1990, Congress heightened it commitment to fund medicaid, but continued to shift a large part of the burden to the states, in ways both more subtle and more daring. It was more subtle in that Congress did not explicitly alter the medicaid

Table 3.4: Comparison of Medicaid and Medicare Reductions in Eligibility and Benefits: 1984 to 1990

Year	Medicaid		Medicare
	Required	Optional	
1984	• restricted eligibility to those who agree to assign to the states any right they had to other health benefits programs		
1985		• permitted states to delete coverage of medically necessary, non-experimental organ transplants	
1986	• eliminated coverage of illegal aliens		
1987			• restricted eligibility for home health care
1989			• repealed virtually all medicare benefits adopted in 1988

Sources: *Congress and the Nation, Vols 6-8; Health Care Financing Review Medicare and Medicaid Statistical Supplement, 1992; Social Security Bulletin,*

matching rate or tighten eligibility for categories of medicaid eligibles, as it had during the earlier period. However, by failing to adequately protect the poor elderly and disabled from gaps in medicare coverage (e.g., the lack of coverage for medications and increasingly onerous medicare cost-sharing requirements), Congress shifted responsibility for health care for these vulnerable populations to the states. Had the federal medicare program been more generously funded, the states would not have had to supplement those benefits through medicaid.

Congress was also more daring between 1984 and 1990 in the extent to which it enacted measures that imposed intrusive and costly requirements upon the states. These included not only dramatic extensions in eligibility and benefits, but requirements to create outstations to recruit new medicaid recipients, to finance the implementation of expensive new quality standards for nursing homes, and to establish a drug rebate program. Although Congress continued to share the cost of these requirements, they represent an unprecedented and unwanted financial toll on the states.

COMPARISON OF MEDICARE AND MEDICAID

Between 1984 and 1990 Congress was not as generous in its treatment of medicare as it was of medicaid. Medicaid became the "darling" of Congress, while medicare, more often than not, suffered budget cuts. (See Table 3.5 for a summary of the difference in congressional treatment of the two programs between 1984 and 1990.) As a result of the many legislated expansions in the medicaid program during the mid and late-1980, enrollment in that program grew from 24.1 million enrollees in 1984 to 31.7 million in 1991 (Holahan 1993, 24). And expenditures likewise increased from $35.5 billion to $87.1 billion in 1991. Its average annual rate of growth equaled 12.5 percent over the last half of the decade, while that of medicare's slowed to 9 percent (*Medicaid Source Book* 1993, 109).

Congress adopted only three expansions in medicare eligibility, and two of them were primarily aimed at increasing revenues for the Hospital Insurance trust fund rather than at expanding the number of those who would be expected to use the benefits immediately. The third made it easier for the previously disabled to resume medicare coverage. These three expansions stand in stark contrast to the magnitude of the

Table 3.5: Comparison of the Numberof Medicaid and Medicare Policy Changes: 1984-1990

Feature	Medicaid		Medicare
	Required	Optional	
Expansion in Eligibility	19	12	3
Expansion in Benefits	11	8	13[1]
Reduction in Eligibility	3	none	1
Reduction in Benefits	none	1	1[2]
Changes in Funding	none[3]	none	13[4]

[1] All of the expansions associated with the 1988 MCCA are counted as only **one** expansion in this figure.

[2] All of the expansions of the 1988 MCCA that were repealed in 1989 are counted as only **one** reduction.

[3] Although no funding changes were required of the states, Congress adopted four provisions that directed HCFA to protect the financial status of the states with regard to matching.funds.

[4] All of the funding changes associated with the MCCA and its repeal are counted as **two changes** in this figure—once when the expansion and its new funding mechanism was enacted, and once when it was repealed.

Sources: *Congress and the Nation,* Vols 2-8; *Social Security Bulletin, Annual Statistical Supplement, 1993.*

expansions in eligibility that Congress awarded poor and near poor pregnant women, children, families, elderly, and aliens during the same period.

Despite the fiscal concerns of the late-1980s, Congress still found it relatively easy to expand benefits for both medicaid and medicare beneficiaries. Although enlargements in the medicaid program have received much attention, medicare's have not been widely noted in the literature. In every year between 1984 and 1990 Congress adopted measures that extended medicare benefits. (See Table 3.3 for greater detail.) It not only enlarged the types of practitioners from whom medicare patients could seek care, but also extended a number of potentially expensive benefits, including a wide variety of out-patient services, liver transplants, hospice benefits, mental health services, osteoporosis treatment, and preventive services such as Pap smears and mammograms. In addition to these incremental extensions in benefits, in 1988, Congress undertook a major expansion in catastrophic benefits in one sweeping bill—the *Medicare Catastrophic Coverage Act (MCCA)*. This measure will be discussed in a separate section below.

Congress demonstrated great reluctance to save money through explicitly reducing benefits to either medicaid or medicare recipients during the late 1980s. Other than repealing the short-lived MCCA in 1989, Congress enacted only one other curtailment in benefits in 1987, when it restricted eligibility for home health care.(See Table 3.4 for a summary of these reductions). Instead of authorizing the elimination of a benefit, Congress preferred to alter the funding arrangements, placing additional responsibilities upon recipients for financing their benefits.

Changes in Medicare Funding

While Congress was busy expanding benefits for medicaid recipients, it looked to medicare for ways to save money. A Congressional Budget Office study concluded that Medicare spending in 1990 was only 82 percent of what it would have been in the absence of legislation to slow its growth rate (CBO 1991). Finding it politically inadvisable to make explicit cutbacks in program benefits or eligibility, Congress focused most of its cost-control efforts on medicare providers. These included placing a freeze on physician payments in 1985 and reforming the reimbursement system for physicians in 1989 to alter incentives so as to promote more conservative primary care rather than expensive, invasive procedures. In addition to these cost-savings measures, others were adopted that concentrated upon home health care and skilled nursing facilities. (See Appendix B for a summary of the major Medicare legislation and provisions).

While it is clear that Congress targeted the providers most directly, essentially all aspects of the program suffered under the congressional knife, according to Marilyn Moon of the Urban Institute. She writes, "Most of the emphasis centered on reducing payments to providers of Medicare services, but beneficiaries also faced reductions in benefits and increased requirements for cost sharing" (1993, 42). She further explains,

> In every budget submission by Presidents Reagan and Bush, proposed cuts in Medicare affecting beneficiaries have constituted a substantial share of the domestic budget reduction agenda. In turn, Congress has included beneficiaries in each of the major budget reduction reconciliation acts, although generally to a lesser degree than the administration has advocated. Thus the elderly and disabled were not immune to the budget cutting of the 1980s (1993, 82).

One of the legislative changes that had a significant impact on medicare beneficiaries arose from a 1982 change in the formula that determined the premium for Part B services. As a result of this measure, beneficiaries shouldered a greater portion of the cost of Part B through higher premiums. The impact was minimal initially, but the provision was revised in 1986 and again in 1990. Moon estimates that in 1991, because of these changes, each beneficiary paid an additional $156 per year—a figure that she predicts will grow faster than the incomes of the elderly and disabled (1993, 84).

Moon has estimated the total direct costs shifted from medicare to its beneficiaries as a result of medicare legislative changes in the 1980s averaged about $210 per enrollee in 1991 (1993, 88). The burden of cost-sharing expenses for covered medicare services more than doubled during the decade of the 1980s. Judith Feder, a health policy expert, explains the significance of this growth. She writes,

> Critics of medicare coverage have frequently observed that the elderly spend as large a share of their incomes on health care today as they did before Medicare was enacted, when spending on noncovered services as well as on cost sharing for covered services is taken into account (1991, 8).

Medicare beneficiaries have been affected not only by the direct costs imposed by legislative changes in the program, but also by the indirect costs. Moon claims that modifications in reimbursement to providers, for example, although difficult to quantify, have had a

Table 3.6: Comparison of Medicaid and Medicare Changes in Funding: 1984-1990

Year	Medicaid		Medicare
	Required	Optional	
1984			• reestablished the provisions that sets the premium for **Part B** at one-fourth the cost of the program for elderly beneficiaries • limited the increase in **Part B** premium to the increase in the COLA for OASDI cash benefits
1984			• reestablished the provisions that sets the premium for **Part B** at one-fourth the cost of the program for elderly beneficiaries • limited the increase in **Part B** premium to the increase in the COLA for OASDI cash benefits
1985			• limited the increase in **Part B** premiums through 1988 to that of the 1986 level

Table 3.6 (continued)

| Year | Medicaid | | Medicare |
	Required	Optional	
1986	• held states harmless as a result of the change from biennial to annual calculation of state matching funds		• extended through 1988 the provisions that sets the premium for **Part B** at one-fourth the cost of the program for elderly beneficiaries • prohibited increase in **Part B** premium if no Social Security COLA • capped 1987 **Part A** deductible at $520, ($52 below what it would have been), and slowed the rate of growth for further increases
1987			• continued (through 1989) to require **Part B** premiums to cover 25% of that program's costs
1988	• established moratorium preventing HHS from publishing final regulations to limit the state's ability to use donated funds through 12/31/89		• increased **Part B** premium for all beneficiaries and established an income-related premium for **Part A**

Table 3.6 (continued)

| Year | Medicaid | | Medicare |
	Required	Optional	
1989	• extended through 12/31/90 the moratorium preventing HHS from publishing final regulations to limit the state's ability to use donated funds		• canceled changes in **Part A** and **Part B** premiums
1990	• extended through 12/31/91 the moratorium preventing HHS from publishing final regulations to limit the state's ability to use donated funds		• raised from $75 to $100 the deductible for **Part B** • continued requiring that beneficiaries of **Part B** pay 25% of the cost of that program through their premiums. • set the rates in advance through 1995, rather than allowing them to float • increased taxable income for HI tax to $125,000 and established a formula for automatic increases in wage base as incomes rise

Sources: *Congress and the Nation*, Vols 6-8; *Social Security Bulletin, Annual Statistical Supplement, 1993.*

significant impact upon beneficiaries. In fact, she claims that some changes induced by the Prospective Payment System (PPS) "may have merely shifted the costs of care onto the beneficiaries or reduced the quality of service as hospitals changed their behavior in response to PPS" (1993, 91).

There is no doubt that Congress allowed an increasing burden of medicare expenditures to fall on beneficiaries, principally through increased cost-sharing, between 1984 and 1990. However, the extent of the congressional effort to devise politically acceptable means of funding the relentlessly growing medicare program has not received much attention. Congress was preoccupied with the funding arrangements for medicare between 1984 and 1990, enacting more changes in those seven years than the preceding nineteen. (See Table 3.6 for a summary of the congressional changes in medicare funding between 1984 and 1990.) It pursued the same three successful strategies that had enabled it to expand medicare so generously during the first 19 years of its existence. It sought to protect medicare beneficiaries from the full impact of rising medicare expenses; it dispersed the costs ever more widely; and when necessary, it increased the costs to beneficiaries very incrementally.

First, although it continued to require that beneficiaries finance one-fourth of the cost of SMI through premiums, it enacted legislation in 1984, 1985, and 1986 that protected beneficiaries from the full impact of this requirement, by mandating that the additional charge for SMI premiums not exceed the dollar amount of the COLA for OASDI beneficiaries. Furthermore, in 1986 Congress capped the deductible for Part A at $520. This figure was $52 below what it would have been under the current law. In addition, Congress altered the formula for determining this charge, slowing its rate of growth.

The second strategy that Congress pursued to minimize opposition to growing medicare costs was to disperse them even more widely. Rather than raising the HI tax rate, which would have subjected low- and middle-income families to an increasing burden, Congress more than doubled the wage base subject to the HI in 1990. The wages subject to that tax rose from $51,300 to $125,000 (See Table 3.7 for the changes in wage base subject to HI).

Table 3.7: Annual Maximum Taxable Earnings and Contribution Rates for Old Age Survivors Insurance and Hospital Insurance: 1984-1991

Date	Annual maximum taxable earnings	Contribution Rate Employer/Employee Each	
		OASI	HI
1984	37,800	5.2 %	1.3 %
1985	39,600	5.2	1.35
1986	42,000	5.2	1.45
1987	43,800	5.2	1.45
1988	45,000	5.53	1.45
1989	48,000	5.53	1.45
1990	51,300	5.6	1.45
1991	125,000	5.6	1.45

Source: U.S. Department of Health and Human Services. 1993. *Annual Supplement, 1993 to the Social Security Bulletin,* 25.

The third way in which Congress raised revenue for medicare, while minimizing opposition, was through ensuring frequent small adjustments in each of the aspects of medicare financing. These included such changes as establishing an automatic mechanism for gradually increasing the Part A deductible and the Part B premium, and enlarging the Part B deductible. (See Table 3.8 for a summary of the changes in medicare cost-sharing between 1984 and 1991.) Congress sought to decrease the impact of these cost increases through assisting those least able to finance them by enlarging medicaid benefits for poor medicare recipients (QMBs). Widespread private medigap insurance coverage and the QMB program for poor medicare recipients helped to diminish the burden of these additional cost-sharing requirements.[2]

Medicare Catastrophic Coverage Act

There was one notable exception to this incremental course of action. In June of 1988 Congress adopted the Medicare Catastrophic Coverage Act (MCCA) amidst great fanfare. This single piece of legislation extended coverage to outpatient drugs and expanded a wide array of other benefits to cover large medical bills so as to limit the financial

Table 3.8: Medicare cost sharing and premium sharing: 1984-1991

Year	Hospital Insurance		Supplementary Medical Insurance		
	Inpatient Hospital Deductible for first 60 days[1]	Monthly Premium for voluntary participation	Annual Deductible[1]	Coinsurance[1]	Monthly Premium for enrollee (aged and disabled)
1984	$356	$174	$75	20%	$14.60
1985	400	214	75	20	15.50
1986	492	226	75	20	15.50
1987	520	234	75	20	17.90
1988	540	156	75	20	24.80
1989	560	175	75	20	31.90
1990	592	177	75	20	28.60
1991	628	177	100	20	29.90

[1]These co-payments do not finance the cost of the program directly, but reflect additional costs to beneficiaries who use HI or SMI benefits.

Source: U.S. Department of Health and Human Services. *Annual Statistical Supplement Social Security Bulletin, 1993*, 87.

risk to medicare beneficiaries. It was hailed as "the largest expansion of Medicare since the program's establishment in 1965" (Torres-Gil 1989, 61), and it was based upon recommendations from the Bowen Commission. That body was charged in the mid 1980s with studying problems associated with catastrophic health expenses, and proposed a rather simple extension in benefits and premium payment by beneficiaries (an increase of $59 per year). However, the legislation that emerged from Congress contained much more expansive benefits and financing.

Unlike the other medicare measures adopted between 1984 and 1990, the MCCA awarded sweeping and expensive benefits—all at once. It provided out-patient drugs, protection for spouses of nursing home residents, limits on out-of-pocket expenses, and improved coverage for home health care and skilled nursing facilities. Such a generous expansion in benefits required an equally sweeping enlargement in funding. Because of the sizable increase in benefits and President Reagan's insistence that financing come from the elderly (rather than taxpayers generally), legislators had to abandon their usual strategy of incrementalism and dispersion. In seeking financing for these new benefits, Congress tried to protect the neediest of the elderly by instituting an income-related Part A premium for the first time. It also enlarged the Part B premium. This had the effect of concentrating the costs on the backs of middle and upper-class elderly. Within a year, opposition to MCCA's funding had solidified among this population of the elderly, and on the last night of the congressional session, November 22, 1989, Congress voted to repeal the MCCA. Moon characterized MCAA as "one of the shortest-lived pieces of social legislation in the United States" (1993, 107). When it repealed this legislation, Congress left intact a very small part of the original bill— those sections which expanded medicaid eligibility for the poor.

CONCLUSION

Between 1984 and 1990, members of Congress deviated from their usual pattern of expanding medicare and curtailing medicaid. They repeatedly and extensively expanded medicaid, imposing sizable costs upon both the states and the federal government in the process. Although Congress also enacted a number of extensions in medicare benefits, their scope and expense did not match those of medicaid.

Rather, the medicare program, especially its providers, became a favorite target of budget cutters in the 1980s. Such a reversal in the congressional treatment of these two programs was highly unexpected and hard to reconcile with conventional understandings of the politics of medicaid.

One important exception to this pattern occurred in 1988. Congress enacted an historic measure that dramatically expanded medicare benefits. However, because of its increased costs, Congress had to devise a new financing mechanism. Rapid and widespread opposition to that funding emerged, forcing Congress to repeal the measure in the following year. The expansions in the medicaid program and the failed extension in medicare illustrate the challenge to policymakers of devising politically acceptable means of program financing during a time of fiscal constraints.

NOTES

1. And, to a lesser extent, it increased the burden upon recipients through cost-sharing.

2. In 1987, 31 percent of the elderly had relatively generous employer-based medigap plans (NCHSR 1989).

CHAPTER FOUR

Medicaid Politics and the Congressional Agenda: 1984 to 1990

Expansion of medicaid reached the congressional agenda in the mid-1980s because the politics of medicaid changed. Medicaid's support grew in breadth and stability between 1984 and 1990. The three attributes that had been weaknesses during its first 19 years were transformed by changing circumstances. Three major developments inside and outside government strengthened medicaid's *political constituency* and *ideological appeal*, and converted its *shared funding* into an asset. Rapidly rising health care costs, growing numbers of the uninsured, and rampant cost-shifting within the health care arena had widespread repercussions throughout society. The scope of these problems helped to generate wide support for expanding federal funding for health care for the poor. Furthermore, a change in the partisan control of Congress during the 1980s also promoted a more liberal agenda. And finally, the prospect of severe and enduring fiscal constraints on the federal government heightened the importance of economic considerations in making policy choices; this increased the significance of medicaid's federal-state shared financing.

John Kingdon's framework suggests that when three *streams* converge—*problem, politics,* and *policy*—the chances of that issue reaching the congressional agenda greatly improve (1984). This describes precisely what occurred in the mid-1980s, prompting Congress to switch its agenda from cutting back medicaid to expanding it. This chapter will examine the factors that led to this change, and show how they bolstered medicaid's support.

WORSENING PROBLEMS IN HEALTH CARE

The relentless growth of health care expenditures as a portion of the federal budget,[1] a conservative mood in the nation, and predictions of insolvency in the medicare HI trust fund brought the issue of health care cost-control to front and center of the congressional agenda in the early 1980s, and prompted members of Congress to institute unprecedented changes in federal health care programs. These included tightening eligibility for AFDC (and therefore, medicaid), reducing the medicaid matching rate for three years, granting states greater flexibility in reimbursing medicaid providers (Boren Amendments), and introducing prospective payment for medicare (PPS). These measures had a major impact on the health care system in this country.

Children were among those most adversely affected by the 1981 medicaid cutbacks. Sally Cohen, health care researcher, writes that in 1983,

> 22 percent of all children were living in poverty—the highest rate in two decades—and the percentage was even higher for children living in black, or single, female-headed households. By 1983, Medicaid covered only 70 percent of poor children, compared to 90 percent in 1979 . . . (231).

As a result of growing concern among various public and private entities during the mid to late 1980s, a number studies highlighting the worsening problems related to access to health care were undertaken. Children were a particular focus of many of these, including one conducted by the task force on infant mortality of the Southern Governors' Association. In the mid 1980s, this study revealed, the southern infant mortality rate was 12.7 deaths per 1000 live births, compared with the national average of 11.5. The South was home to ten of the 11 states with the highest infant mortality rates (Kosterlitz 1986, 2258). An impressive array of statistics also exhibited deteriorating health indicators for infants and young children throughout the nation during the 1980s, including such areas as prenatal care, low birthweight, infant mortality, and childhood immunization status (Rosenbaum 1993a, 50).

Children were not the only group affected, however. The number of uninsured also grew during the 1980s, in part because of federal actions. Socioeconomic factors, such as the three recessions of that decade and changes in employment from heavy manufacturing to service industries also contributed to increasing their ranks. Between 1980 and 1987 the number of uninsured increased by 25 percent to 37 million (Fraser 1991, 302).[2] Even for many who were fortunate enough to possess insurance during this period, coverage was often inadequate when compared with their medical expenses. Although agreement on the definition of *underinsured* is lacking, estimates suggest that from 8 to 26 percent of those under 65 with private insurance were underinsured in the early 1980s (Farley 1985, 477). Because of rampant cost-shifting, growth in the number of uninsured and underinsured affected a broad spectrum of interests, such as health care providers, insurers, and purchasers of insurance (including employers), as well state and local governments.

Hospitals, where the bulk of uncompensated care occurs, were especially affected by the simultaneous impact of rising numbers of uninsured and tightening of public and private reimbursement (Cohodes 1986, 228). Prior to some of the most stringent cost-cutting measures, many hospitals were already experiencing fiscal difficulty. Not all hospitals were equally in a position to absorb the cost of charity care, nor was the distribution of charity care equal among all hospitals. Judy Feder writes,

> In 1980, most short-term general, non-federal, non-profit hospitals were in reasonably good financial health . . . Private teaching hospitals and public hospitals outside the 100 largest cities shared in this good health . . . While most hospitals did well, some hospitals had serious fiscal problems; almost one-quarter lost money in 1980 . . . In metropolitan areas, especially the largest cities, stress resulted largely from extensive care to the poor . . . combined with insufficient revenues from either private-insured patients or government sources to finance that care (1984, 238-239).

This problem worsened during the 1980s. The American Hospital Association reported that the amount of uncompensated care delivered by hospitals rose dramatically from $3.5 billion in 1980 to nearly $9 billion in 1987 (Fraser 1991, 304). As a percentage of all community hospital revenues, uncompensated care climbed from 6.2 percent in 1980 to 9.1 percent in 1990. The burden on state and local hospitals was even greater, with uncompensated care costs increasing from 14.3 to 18.8 percent of revenues over the same period (Letsch 1992, 12). Physicians also delivered a sizable amount of unreimbursed care, estimated to be $2.9 billion in 1982 (Cohodes 1986, 229).

Cutbacks in medicare reimbursement only worsened the financial strain on hospitals. Examining data from 1983 to 1990, Marilyn Moon of the Urban Institute writes,

> Many hospitals are finding it more difficult to cover the costs of providing care to [medicare] beneficiaries. Frequently hospitals have not acted aggressively to hold down costs of care. Consequently, they must either face losses or find ways to shift costs onto other groups paying for hospital care (such as patients covered by private insurance) (1993, 59).

This problem was widespread. The *Wall Street Journal* reported in 1991, that "more than half of U.S. hospitals will lose money on medicare this year" (Marchasin 1991).

In order to recover those losses, health care providers inflate the cost to the privately insured, since 73.2 percent of the population had such coverage. One estimate suggests that cost-shifting from the uninsured, medicaid, medicare, and discounted managed care plans added 67 percent to health insurance for indemnity plans in 1990 (Department of Political Science, Northeastern University hereafter DPSNEU 1994, 14). Sidney Marchasin, the chairman of the board of Sequoia Hospital in Redwood City, California reported the extent of his institution's cost-shifting to private insurance companies. He explained,

> Indemnity plans (i.e., commercial insurance companies that pay the hospital's usual fee for each item of service) are bearing the brunt of the cost shift. Between 1989 and 1991, trying to make up for our $26 million loss from medicare and medicaid, Sequoia charged commercial insurers $24 million more than the actual costs of its services (1991).

Business, the largest purchaser of private insurance, has been at the end of the cost-shifting cycle. Along with their employees, they have born a large portion of the burden of uninsured and decreased public spending on health care. Employer contributions to employee health insurance premiums swelled by 352 percent between 1970 and 1989, due in large part to cost-shifting among payers. Corporate health spending reached $173.4 billion in 1989, and then increased further, by 21.6 percent in 1990, according to researchers at Northeastern University (DPSNEU 1994, 14). Cohodes describes the sentiment of the business community as follows:

> Business has an enormous vested interest in assuring that insurance protection is widespread. Increasingly, business has come to realize that it is financing the costs of care that no one else wished to underwrite. In effect, and inadvertantly, business has supplanted government as the payer of last resort for those who fall between the gaps of private and public insurance. Business, not surprisingly would like to reduce its burden (1986, 231).

This country has historically been more tolerant of high health care expenditures and large numbers of uninsured than other western nations; however, these problems worsened significantly during the mid-1980s. The fact that many of these difficulties emerged as the result of earlier public policies, (e.g., cutbacks in AFDC eligibility and reductions in medicare reimbursements to providers), increased the perception that they were legitimate issues for government to address. Furthermore, their persistence throughout the 1980s further explains, not only how they emerged on the congressional agenda, but why they remained high on the list of congressional priorities for seven years.

CHANGE IN POLITICAL SUPPORT

In contrast to the years between 1965 and 1983 when medicaid's political support was weak, the level of political support for expanding medicaid remained quite strong and consistent between 1984 and 1990. Medicaid's popularity was stronger in part because of its increased importance as a source of federal health care financing to a broad array of groups. Consequently, support in Congress did not wane as the states grew increasingly resistant to mandatory extensions in that program.

This broad support was seen in the very first piece of expansionary legislation, enacted in 1984. Alice Sardell, health policy analyst, describes the coalition supporting that expansion. She writes,

> A broad coalition of groups worked to enact this legislation, including the children's Defense Fund, the American Academy of Pediatrics, the March of Dimes, the National Association of Community Health Centers, the Association of Maternal and Child Health Programs, the Catholic Conference, and the National Governors' Association. Conservative, right-to life members of Congress and some corporate business leaders also were supportive (1991, 28).

Support for the expansion of medicaid had two fundamental bases: *ideological* and *distributional*. The number of those supporting an expansion of health care for the poor because of ideological reasons increased during the 1980s. Furthermore, the many health care groups benefiting from an addition of public funding for the uninsured also became more visible and vocal.

Ideological support grew stronger because of two main factors. First, elections favored Democrats, increasing their numbers in Congress during the 1980s. This altered the congressional agenda in a decidedly more liberal direction (Ferejohn 1991). And second, advocates for the poor worked hard to re-shape and broaden the ideological appeal of expanding health care for poor children (Sardell 1991, Cohen 1991).

The partisan composition of Congress played a major role in altering the agenda of the 1980s (Ferejohn, 1991). (See Table 4.1 for a breakdown of partisan composition during the 1980s). Because welfare programs are generally very dependent upon ideological appeal for their political support, this view suggests they are particularly susceptible to electoral changes. Therefore, as Congress became increasingly Democratic, restorations of social welfare programs for the poor became more likely. Until 1987, Congress remained divided, with a Democratic House and Republican Senate. Although the Democrats remained in control of the House throughout the period, their electoral success was mixed. The most crucial electoral change occurred in 1986 when elections brought an end to Republican control of the Senate. Controlling both houses meant Democrats were better positioned to shape the congressional agenda, and the emergence of a consensus for the reform of social policies was more likely (Cohen 1991, 231-232).

Health care was an issue that captured the attention of congressional Democrats in the 1980s. They were instrumental in bringing attention to problems related to health care through holding hearings, sponsoring studies on children's health, and creating a special

Table 4.1: Party Control of the Senate and House: 1979 - 1991

Congress	Years	Senate			House		
		D	R	I	D	R	I
96th	1979-1981	58	41	1	276	157	-
97th	1981-1983	46	53	1	243	192	-
98th	1983-1985	45	55	-	267	168	-
99th	1985-1987	47	53	-	252	183	-
100th	1987-1989	55	45	-	258	177	-
101st	1989-1991	55	45	-	260	175	-

Source: Davidson, Roger H. And Walter J. Oleszek. 1994. *Congress and Its Members.* 4th ed. Washington, D.C.: Congressional Quarterly.

committee—the House Select Committee on Children, Youth and Families in 1982. Their increased control after 1986 helps to explain why Democrats in Congress succeeded in enacting some of the most expansive medicaid measures during the later years of the decade. Expansions adopted during the mid-1980s, when control of Congress was less firmly in Democratic hands, tended to be more optional and less intrusive than those adopted later. (See Table 3.1 and 3.3 for a comparison of optional and required extensions in the medicaid program between 1984 and 1990).

Partisan influence has not generally been a dominant factor in medicaid policymaking, however. Rosenbaum reminds us that, "Between 1977 and 1980, a Democratic President and a Democratic Congress twice tried and twice failed, to enact legislation covering only a portion of the pregnant women and children aided during the 1980s" (1993a, 47). Other factors besides a liberal Congress were instrumental in building strong support for medicaid.

Much credit belongs to advocates of the poor for building stronger ideological support for the medicaid program. Having failed to win sufficient support in the late 1970s and early 1980s, they were more determined and more skilled in persuading other to support enlarging federal funding for the poor in the later 1980s. Alice Sardell explicitly cites "the failure of advocates to use the media to arouse the public on children's health issues" and "the lack of a perceived crisis" as major factors in the downfall of attempts in the 1970s to expand medicaid (1991, 26-27). The child health advocates in the 1980s learned from those lessons.

One way in which they built support was through publicizing the disturbing trends in children's health. Cohen claims:

> Congressional support for medicaid was not strong enough to prevent these cuts [1980-1983] until child health advocates organized lobbying efforts and presented the dismal facts of deteriorating maternal and child health to Congress and the public. From 1983 to 1989 soaring infant mortality rates, among other factors, became a national embarrassment and goaded lawmakers into passing landmark legislation restoring the cutbacks of the earlier part of the decade (1991, 229).

They helped to fund private research and publicize the results of those studies and of government research that revealed the deteriorating status of children's health.

Second, they framed the issue of children's health in such a way as to appeal broadly to American values. Instead of framing the issue simply as a *liberal* welfare matter, advocates sought to win mainstream support (Sardell, 1991, 31). Although American social policy has a bias toward the elderly, the *New York Times* reports that American voters are more willing to help other people's children than other (non-elderly) adults, especially when race is involved (Dionne 1987, 36). Sardell elucidates the values that advocates emphasized, including: pragmatism (childhood problems are preventable and therefore amenable to solution); cost-effectiveness (preventing childhood problems saves money in the long run); investment in the future (children are import for the future success of the U.S. economy); and children as innocent victims (children are morally blameless for their condition) (1991, 31-35).

Medicaid's distribution of benefits to a broad constituency provided a second basis for that program's unusually high level of support during the mid- to late-1980s. Ferejohn argues that the wide distribution of benefits, not ideological appeal, is what provides medicaid advantages over other, more narrowly focused welfare programs. He states, "One way to reduce the divisiveness of a policy proposal is to ensure that its benefits are very widely distributed" (1991, 130). Differentiating among types of social welfare policies and their respective levels of support, Ferejohn writes,

> In effect, these various political arrangements have yielded three kinds of programs: programs that are politically popular (even untouchable) but very inefficient at transferring income to the "truly needy"; programs that are relatively efficient in this regard but which are politically vulnerable; and programs that are supported by an alliance of producers and clients, which share benefits between these groups and transfer income to the poor at the cost of subsidizing relatively high income producers (1991, 130).

Medicaid falls into his third category. Over time, as federal sources of health care financing shrunk, medicaid funds became increasingly important to a wide variety of participants in the health care world—producers, insurers, purchasers of insurance, and clients.

These groups organized the Children's Medicaid Coalition during the late 1980s. Robert Pear, reporter for the *New York Times*, remarks on the surprisingly diverse membership in this coalition. He writes,

> The United States Chamber of Commerce does not normally lobby for poor children. Nor does the National Association of Manufacturers usually advocate expansion of government programs (1990).

However, according to Pear, these two groups, along with, "doctors, hospitals, health insurers and advocates for children" organized the coalition to "persuade Congress to expand Medicaid . . . " (1990).

The Chamber of Commerce declared, "Poor children are not a natural constituency of ours. But it is important to the business community to have a healthy productive work force . . . " The National Association of Manufacturers proclaimed that the expansion of medicaid "makes good business sense." And a representative of the Metropolitan Life Insurance Company stated, "It is an unfair tax on our policyholders . . . for them to have to bear the burden of paying for people who are poor and unable to buy their own insurance." Fear of greater government intervention was also a motivation. A representative of the health insurance industry remarked, "If we don't find a way to provide coverage for the nation's 31 million uninsured, the Federal Government may move to adopt some foolish, ill-advised, ill-conceived national health insurance strategy." Pear concludes that these members were motivated by "a combination of altruism and financial self-interest" (1990, 24).

Although support for medicaid expansion remained unusually strong and united during the 1984 to 1990 years, one important group jumped ship. During the mid-1980s states were among those advocating optional expansions in the medicaid program, but they soon became the strongest opponent of the congressional expansions. Initially states sought to loosen the medicaid eligibility rules that would allow them to de-couple medicaid and AFDC. Such a change would permit them to extend medicaid coverage and received federal matching funds for previously excluded groups, (e.g., two-parent families and the near-poor) while not having to extend AFDC to these populations. Congress welcomed state support for expansions, but instead of granting states the option of expanding their programs, it delivered a string of mandatory medicaid requirements. The financial burden of these mandates produced an outcry among the states in congressional hearings on medicaid during the late 1980s. Appealing publicly to Congress in 1989, 49 of the 50 governors sought an end to further required medicaid expansions. However, given the broad support and momentum for expansions, Congress ignored them.

FISCAL CONSTRAINTS

The first two circumstances, worsening problems in the health care sector and a rise in political support for enlarging health care programs for the poor, help to explain why members of Congress changed their priorities in the mid-1980s from cutting to expanding funding for this population. In addition, the severity of the federal government's financial circumstances helped medicaid to win out as the most appealing policy alternative. While fiscal concerns always exert some influence over congressional policymaking, the depth of the federal deficit, long-term projections for rising entitlement expenses, and the anti-tax sentiment among the public during the 1980s heightened the importance of economic considerations at this time.

The fiscal condition of the federal government became much worse in the early 1980s. A number of factors contributed to the federal deficit, including a tax cut in 1981, a rapidly aging society, and the growing portion of the federal budget that was committed to entitlements for the elderly. The deficit climbed from $79 billion in 1981 to $207.8 billion in 1983 and hovered near there for the rest of the decade (*Economic Report of the President* 1994, 359). (See Figure 4.1 for a comparison of the deficit during the 1980s with that of earlier decades). The anti-tax sentiment of the public during the 1980s also presented a major obstacle to reducing that figure. This fiscal context limited the congressional agenda and heightened the importance of program costs when considering policy alternatives.

While Congress might have selected any number of other programs to expand health care coverage for the poor during this decade, including the Maternal and Child Health Block Grant, the Community Migrant Health Centers and Infant Mortality Initiative, and the National Service Corps, it did not. These were never seriously considered. Weiner and Engle compare the growth rates for these programs with that of medicaid (1991, 48). Each one either failed to keep up with the medical inflation rate or suffered actual reductions in its absolute growth during the 1980s. (See Table 4.2 for a description of the growth of various programs during the 1980s).

Medicare might also have been used as a vehicle for expanding federal health care financing to the needy, or at least to some of the needier medicare recipients. The elderly are a large and well-organized constituency that made a strong claim in the 1980s that medicare benefits were inadequate.[3] Congress employed two main strategies to extend benefits to this needy population. One involved expanding benefits for poor medicare recipients through extensions in the medicaid program (i.e., the QMB program). This approach shifted part of the cost of enlargements to the states. The second strategy, the MCCA of 1988, involved enlarging medicare and having the elderly finance the cost of the program according to an income-related premium.

While Congress's first approach, extending benefits for the elderly through the medicaid program, remained intact, and was even expanded in 1990, Congress was forced to repeal nearly all the provisions of the

Figure 4.1: Average Deficit by Decade

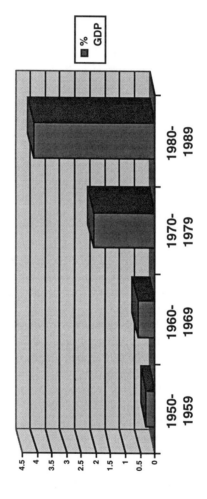

Source: General Accounting Office.1990. *The Budget Deficit: Outlook, Implications, and Choices.* Washington, D.C.: Government Printing Office, 3.

Table 4.2: Federal Appropriations and Expenditures for Selected Health Programs, FY 1980 to 1990 (millions of dollars)

Year	Maternal and child health block grant	Community/ migrant health centers and infant mortality initiative	National Health Service Corps	Total	Medicaid	Medical consumer price index
1980	433	360	154	947	14,000	74.9
1981	455	367	148	970	16,800	82.9
1982	374	319	131	824	17,400	92.5
1983	478	398	104	980	19,000	100.6
1984	399	393	74	866	20,100	106.8
1985	478	427	48	953	22,700	113.5
1986	457	441	58	956	25,000	122.0
1987	497	465	42	1,004	27,400	130.1
1988	527	459	43	1,029	30,500	138.6
1989	554	481	48	1,083	34,600	149.3
1990	554	506	51	1,111	41,100	161.9
Average annual compound rate of growth (percent)	2.5	3.5	-10.5	1.6	11.3	8.0

Source: Weiner, Joshua M. and Jeannie Engel. 1991. *Improving Access to Health Services for Children and Pregnant Women*. Washington, D.C.: The Brookings Institution, 48.

MCCA the year after its enactment. The costs of the first approach fell to a group that was unable to influence the electoral success of members of Congress, whereas the costs of the second approach fell squarely upon the shoulders of one of the largest and most well-organized voting blocks in society.[4]

Under the fiscal cloud of the mid- and late-1980s, medicaid's shared financing with the states was transformed from a weakness into an asset. Whereas this sharing of costs with the states had promoted strong state opposition to mandatory aspects of medicaid in the 1960s and 1970s, sharing now had a heretofore underappreciated advantage for congressional policymakers seeking to extend benefits.

Although medicaid's flexibility, multiple missions, and targeting of the poor have been suggested as reasons why it was such a logical choice for expanding health care financing for the poor (Rosenbaum 1993a, 46), these were not its most significant attributes. Without its shared funding, extensive and repeated enlargements in the medicaid program would have been unlikely.

Although advocates tried to expand this program through full federal funding, Congress proved unwilling. In the late 1970s legislation to have the federal government assume 100 percent of the cost of expansions in medicaid was considered and defeated. It was proposed again in 1984 with the states' full support, but it again failed.[5] Henry Waxman, (D-CA), chair of the Subcommittee for Health and the Environment of the House Energy and Commerce Committee faced off with Senator Robert Dole, (R-KA) in the conference committee negotiations over this issue. It became clear that in order to win the support of the Republican Senate for medicaid expansions, this idea would have to be dropped. When Waxman switched the proposal to a shared financing strategy, it saved the federal government millions of dollars and eventually passed both Houses of Congress (Demkovich 1984, 1311). This illustration reveals the significance of shared funding to the acceptance of medicaid as a strategy.

Sharing costs with the states offered Congress two major advantages that helped make medicaid their consistent choice for expansions to the needy during the mid-to late 1980s. First, it was more economically efficient (Schlesinger and Kronebusch 1990, 94). Because the federal government financed only about half of the costs of the medicaid program, expanding it gave the members of Congress more bang for the buck. And second, it provided the most politically acceptable means of dispersing the costs associated with the expansions. Under strong pressure to expand public health care financing for the poor and near-poor, Congress found it easier to consider expanding a program that distributed half the cost to the states rather than to voting entities. This approach permitted members of Congress to claim credit for providing benefits to a wide range of groups, while permitting members to avoid considering the full financial impact of their decision.

CONCLUSION

Although Congress had cut medicaid in the early 1980s, developments inside and outside government strengthened that program's *political constituency* and *ideological appeal*, and transformed its *shared funding* into an asset. Worsening problems in the health care arena and political changes that favored medicaid stimulated pressure for Congress to increase federal financing of health care. In the context of serious fiscal pressures at the federal level in the late 1980s, medicaid's federal-state shared financing status, which had contributed to its political instability in the 1970s, provided it political and fiscal advantagesthat made it the most appealing alternative. Enlarging benefits to a broad constituency, while shifting part of the cost to the states, proved an irresistible strategy for members of Congress. Expanding medicaid emerged because of the special circumstances that highlighted the appeal of that policy. It remained on the agenda for seven years because those circumstances persisted.

The changing circumstances discussed above illuminate why the expansion of medicaid captured and held the attention of Congress during the mid- to late 1980s. However, they do not explain the extent of the enlargements in that program, or how advocates managed to overcome the roadblocks to adoption, not just once, but repeatedly. Had it not been for institutional changes, an alteration in the norms of *federalism* and in the *congressional budget process*, as well as the persistence of a highly skilled policy *entrepreneur*, Rep. Henry Waxman (D-CA), the scope of medicaid's enlargement would certainly have been much smaller. The next three chapters address these developments and analyze how they helped to promote the repeated adoption of enlargements in the medicaid program.

NOTES

1. As a percentage of total government expenditures, federal health care expenditures rose from 3.9 percent in 1965 to 11.7 percent in 1980 (Letsch et al. 1992, 8).

2. The percentage of uninsured persons in the U.S. population increased from 14.9 in 1980 to 17.4 in 1990 (Levit 1992, 35).

3. Because of rapidly rising health care expenditures and the increasing gaps in medicare coverage, the out-of-pocket costs of the elderly reached an unprecedented portion of their incomes in the late 1980s (Moon 1993, 10-11).

4. Even though a relatively small portion of the elderly would pay the maximum tax, a groundswell of opposition emerged among the elderly, fanned by the rhetoric of the National Committee to Protect Social Security (Moon 1993, 124).

5. Waxman also attempted unsuccessfully to increase the federal matching rate to finance extensions in medicaid in both 1990 and 1991.

CHAPTER FIVE

Changes in Institutions: Federalism

Despite the convergence of events in the mid-1980s that brought medicaid expansions to the congressional agenda, the adoption of that policy was by no means guaranteed. Even less certain was the enactment of a succession of these. Political, fiscal, and institutional obstacles existed that might have prevented any extension of medicaid, or at least limited its scope. The decentralized congressional policymaking system and divided government, with separate branches controlled by different parties, frequently led to stalemate. Large budget deficits and anti-big government sentiment limited the ability of Congress to make any program enlargements in the 1980s. Furthermore, the opposition of President Ronald Reagan and fiscal conservatives in Congress, as well as unified and passionate pleas from the states to stop medicaid mandates, might have been fatal. However, due to some important institutional developments and the determination of a very skillful policy entrepreneur, Congress repeatedly overcame these impediments.

CONGRESSIONAL COMMANDS: MEDICAID 1984 - 1990

Carried out through a series of congressional mandates upon the states, the expansion of medicaid was an extreme example of the heightened use of federal power in intergovernmental relations. These measures were intrusive, imposed a sizable fiscal burden, and occurred despite the states' strong opposition. The mandates dictated encompassing standards for eligibility and benefits, and extended far beyond the scope of earlier welfare measures. These included the requirement that states implement new standards for certifying and measuring the performance of long term care facilities *and* that states finance the cost to the facilities of complying with them. Furthermore, instead of allowing states discretion over reimbursement, Congress required them to augment payments to Disproportionate Share Hospitals (DSH). It also ordered states to establish additional, more convenient, locations (e.g., including DSHs and federally qualified health centers) for recipients to apply for medicaid; and commanded them to make the application forms more easily understood so as to facilitate that process. From 1984 to 1990, the cost of medicaid to state and local governments rose from $23.3 billion to $33 billion (in constant dollars) (Coughlin et al. 1994a, 15). As a portion of state budgets, this growth represented an increase from 10 percent in 1984 to nearly 15 percent in 1990 (Burke 1991, 35).

In 1989 the states mounted a public and remarkably unified appeal to Congress to stop. First, Raymond C. Scheppach, Executive Director of the NGA protested to the Senate Finance Committee in June 1989:

> By enacting new mandates, Congress is failing to recognize the fiscal environments in which states operate . . . Trying to deal with such a large and growing program expense at the state level, where budgets must be balanced each year, is not an easy task. The task becomes much more difficult if the flexibility in program design is taken out of the states' hands (SFC Hearing 1989, 215).

Meanwhile, the House proceeded to approve a package of generous medicaid expansions. In response, 49 governors voted for an NGA resolution requesting a two-year moratorium on such measures.[1] James Martin, legislative counsel for the NGA, remarked that in twenty years, he had never seen the states "more unified on any issue" (1995). Several governors testified before Congress and many lobbied their state congressional delegations that summer and fall—to no avail. In October of that year, Congress adopted medicaid expansions that were expected to cost nearly $1 billion by 1991 (Kirschten 1989, 3044-3045).

Many governors and intergovernmental interest groups continued to oppose expansions vociferously throughout the 1990s despite the political pressure and criticism from congressional Democrats, led by Rep. Henry Waxman. In 1990 The National Conference of State Legislatures, sent Congress a letter requesting a halt in medicaid mandates (Coughlin et al. 1994a, 81). These efforts were also in vain.

Some of the most sweeping mandates were adopted in that year. Congress's repeated actions, despite clear and resolute appeals from the states to stop, represents a departure from its earlier, more cooperative relationship with the states.

CHANGES IN FEDERALISM

Such action could not have occurred but for the increase in federal intrusion generally. The term *mandates* came into common usage in the language of intergovernmental relations in the early 1980s, having been introduced by Edward I. Koch in an article, "The Mandate Millstone" (1980). Since then, much attention has focused upon the federal government's increasing intrusiveness in relation to the states. The mandated extensions in the medicaid program reflect the changing nature of the federal-state relationship.

These developments did not begin during the 1980s. Profound changes were already underway in federal-state relations in the mid 1960s when the original medicaid statute was adopted. The 1965 medicaid legislation exemplified them. The 1954 Supreme Court decision, *Brown v. Board of Education*, and various successor decisions on school desegregation marked a sea-change in the customs of federal-state relations. Historically, the Supreme Court had interpreted the Constitution to impose prohibitions on the states.[2] In describing the court in that earlier era, constitutional law scholar Henry M. Hart wrote, "it is illuminating to observe how rarely [the federal court] says, Do *this* thing . . . "(1955, 194). *Brown v. Board of Education* signified the start of an era in which the federal government issued affirmative commands to the states, not merely prohibitions. No longer treating the states as an independent, co-equal level of government, the federal government has become both more commanding and more intrusive (ACIR 1984, 1).

Instead of relying upon the carrot of federal grants and conditions-of-aid to gain state cooperation, the federal government has relied increasingly upon sticks of various sorts, including legislative regulation, preemption, and judicial decrees. The Advisory Commission on Intergovernmental Relations (ACIR) concludes that with these newer strategies, "compliance has been made difficult to avoid" (1984, 7).

These mandates have affected such traditional areas of state autonomy as public employment practices, accessibility to public transit systems, conditions of prisons and jails, speed limits, and availability of public education for handicapped children (ACIR 1984, 2). A number of criticisms have emerged as the scope of federal intrusion has increased. Analysts have argued that the growth of federal regulations places a tremendous fiscal burden on states and their subdivisions without their input, violating important republican principles (ACIR 1984, 47; Derthick 1992, 53). Others hold that commanding states to conform to federal standards discourages diversity and innovation among states. Some critics cite the inefficiency and ineffectiveness of applying national solutions to local jurisdictions without regard for particular circumstances (Koch, 1980). Increasingly, scholars have asserted that the states in many respects have been reduced to "mere agents" of the federal government (Derthick 1992, 52).

THE MEDICAID EXAMPLE

Medicaid was framed when the practice of heightened command was developing. The Social Security Amendments of 1965 that produced medicaid are remarkable for the extent to which they differ from their two predecessors—the Amendments in 1950 that introduced the principle of funding medical vendor payments for recipients of public assistance and those Amendments in 1960 that created the medical assistance program for the elderly known as Kerr-Mills. A comparison of these three measures reveals a progression in the quantity and intrusiveness of the conditions-of-aid that Congress imposed. While it required only three pages to lay out the statutes associated with the 1950 vendor payment program, it took six pages for the 1960 medical assistance amendments, and ten for the 1965 Amendments that established medicaid. (See Table 5. 1 for a summary of the provisions of these three measures).

In 1950, Congress authorized paying providers (vendors) directly for the health care expenses of the poor. The scope of this legislation and the conditions it imposed upon the states were relatively limited. It prescribed standard administrative requirements, (e.g., establishing a single state agency, reporting, and providing for a fair hearing).[3] Although eligibility was limited to those qualifying for cash assistance under one of the Titles of the Social Security Act (OAA, AB, ATPD,

Table 5.1 Comparison of Requirements of Social Security Amendments: 1950, 1960, and 1965

	1950	1960	1965
Administrative Requirements	• Provide the plan is in effect in all sub-divisions of the state	• Same	• Same
	• Financial participation by the state	• Same	• State will pay not less that 40% of non-federal share; effective 7/1/70 state must pay full non-federal share or if not, ensure equal services throughout the state
	• Establish single state agency	• Same	• Same, plus required that determination of eligibility be made by be made by agency determining OASDI eligibility
	• Ensure a fair hearing for those denied	• Same	• Same
	• Provide administration necessary for proper and efficient operation	• Same	• Same

Table 5.1 (continued)

	1950	1960	1965
Administrative Requirements (cont.)			
	Make and verify reports as required	Same	Same
	Provide that no recipient receives aid under more than one program (OAA, AB, ATPD, ADC)	Same	Same
	Provide safeguards regarding disclosure of information	Same	Same
	Provide opportunity for all wishing to make application	Same	Same
	For payments to institutions, establish a State authority to establish and maintain standards	Same	Same

Table 5.1 (continued)

	1950	1960	1965
Eligibility	Eligibility under one of the cash assistance programs: OAA, AB, ATPD, ADC	Created new category of eligible: Medical Assistance for the Aged (MAA)--not recipients of OAA, but for those 65 years of age or over, whose income and resources are insufficient to meet the costs of necessary medical services[1]	Extended coverage to those eligible for AB, ATPD, and ADC and children not receiving cash benefits and complex categories of the medically needy related to those categories as well as two groups of non-categorically related
	In determining need, shall consider any other income and resources	Include reasonable standards for determining eligibility and the extent of aid	Same, and establish comparable standards for all groups, and it limited the inclusion of income and resources

Table 5.1 (continued)

	1950	1960	1965
Eligibility (cont.)	May not impose residence requirement, stricter than: has lived in the state for 5 of the last 9 years and has lived within the state continuously for the past one year	May not impose any residency requirement (except current resident) and the state must provide for the inclusion of state residents who are absent	Same
	Excludes inmates of public institutions (Except medical institutions) (Excludes TB and mentally ill patients in any institution)	Amends to permit payment to medical institutions for mentally ill or TB patients for the first 42 days of care for these diseases	Permits coverage of instiutionalized mentally ill and those with TB over 65 years
	Not applicable	Prohibits enrollment fee, premium or similar charge	Prohibits no deduction or cost sharing for in-patient care; any other charges must be reasonably related to income and resources of recipients

Table 5.1 (continued)

	1950	1960	1965
Eligibility (cont.)			• Must establish safeguards to assure eligibility will be determined and care and services provided in a manner consistent with simplicity of administration and in the best interest of the recipient
Services	• Provides the state the option to finance all or any portion of medical care or any type of remedial care recognized under State law	• Must provide for inclusion of some institutional and non-institutional care and services; may include payment for all or part of the cost of care for 11 different categories of services listed, or any other medical care or remedial care recognized under state law	• Same, and effective 7/1/67, states must provide: in-patient and out-patient hospital services, laboratory and x-ray services, skilled nursing home services, and MD services

Table 5.1 (continued)

	1950	1960	1965
Services (continued)			Set payment method to cover reasonable costs of in-patient services
			For states having mental health provisions for those over 65 years, set extensive requirements for coverage
			For poor medicare recipients, must pay deductible for Part A and income-related assistance with other cost-sharing requirements of that program

Table 5.1 (continued)

	1950	1960	1965
Services (continued)			States required to make efforts toward *broadening the scope of the care and services* and in the direction of *liberalizing the eligibility requirements with a view of furnishing comprehensive care and services to all individuals who meet eligibility standards by 7/1/75*
Financing	Matching grants to states for vendor payments	More generous matching federal and state; federal share ranges between 50% and 80% based on state per capita income	Even more generous matching rates ranging from 55% to 83%, based upon per capita income of state

Table 5.1 (continued)

	1950	1960	1965
Financing (continued)	Complex sharing formula that sets limits on individual and total payments	No limits on individual payments or total state expenditure	Same
		Prohibit liens against property except after death of individual and spouse	Same and expanded to include exceptions: no lien until a surviving child reaches 21, or if child is blind or disabled
			Provide 75% federal matching funds for skilled medical professionals hired to administer the plan and 50% for other administration costs
			States must maintain their effort in funding this program when compared to previous years or suffer a reduced matching rate

[1] In 1962 a similar category of Blind and Totally and Permanently Disabled whose incomes and resources exceeded the limits for cash assistance were also created.

ADC), states retained discretion regarding income, resource, and residency requirements. The law also permitted the states complete control over the type and amount of health care services they would provide. A complex matching formula was less generous than later measures (Social Security Amendments, hereafter SSA 1950).

Given the rising costs of health care, the inadequacy of the earlier plan, and growing concern for the elderly, Congress expanded health care financing for that population in 1960. Although this legislation provided a more generous matching formula to entice state participation,[4] it also contained more stringent requirements. This measure created a new category of eligibility, the near-poor elderly.[5] It also sharply limited state discretion regarding eligibility, prohibiting states from establishing any residency requirements and requiring them to provide for absent residents. Unlike the earlier measure, this statute explicitly forbid states from requiring beneficiaries to pay any enrollment fee or premium for participation. Liens against the property of a beneficiary prior to the death of the beneficiary and her spouse for any purpose related to this program were also prohibited. Furthermore, although the law still allowed states great discretion in the amount and type of care they paid for, it offered a greater degree of specificity than in 1950, stating that states must finance both *institutional and non-institutional care and services* (SSA 1960).

The 1965 Social Security Amendments, which created the medicare and medicaid programs, incorporated even more stringent conditions-of-aid for the states. Although participation in medicaid was optional, Congress strengthened the incentives to participate by phasing out payments under the Kerr-Mills program. Some of the new statutory requirements included:

Financing—The medicaid program provided a slightly more generous matching formula for states, ranging from 55 percent to 83 percent, depending upon the states' per capita income. Whereas states had relied heavily upon local governments for financing the non-federal share of the Kerr-Mills program,[6] this measure required states to fund 40 percent of the non-federal share. Furthermore, Congress established a deadline of July 1, 1970 for each state to pay the full, non-federal share or to ensure that an equal level of services existed throughout that state. It also required states to maintain the level of financing effort that they had made under Kerr-Mills.

Eligibility—The 1965 statute required states to extend coverage to specified groups of individuals, and it allowed them to provide coverage to certain others. The exact nature of these requirements was enshrouded in "the murkiest language of Title XIX," according to Stevens and Stevens (1974, 61). Administrators had difficulty in translating the statutes into comprehensible regulations; in the end they created four separate categories of eligibility, including: the *categorically needy, categorically related needy, categorically related medically needy,* and the *noncategorically related medically needy.* These categories encompassed a much broader range of eligibles than had been previously permitted. The statute also instituted restrictions on the income and resources the states could consider when determining eligibility.

Services—This measure went much farther than earlier ones. It stipulated that states must provide a minimum of five types of services. It also dictated that states pay for the cost-sharing requirements associated with the new medicare program (e.g., the deductible for part A) for their poor elderly, blind, and disabled. However, the most far-reaching condition was the requirement that states enlarge the scope of their programs over time. Section 1903 (e) reads:

> The Secretary shall not make payments under the preceding provisions of this section to any State unless the State makes a satisfactory showing that it is making **efforts in the direction of broadening the scope of the care and services** made available under the plan and **in the direction of liberalizing the eligibility requirements** for medical assistance, with a view toward **furnishing by July 1, 1975, comprehensive care and services to substantially all individuals who meet the plan's eligibility standards** . . . (emphasis mine) (SSA 1965).

Mandating such extensions, complete with a deadline, boldly undermined the long-standing principle that states possess discretion in matters related to the generosity of their welfare programs.

Another requirement that circumscribed state discretion and imposed a hardship upon state governments over the next decade was one that mandated the use of a particular form of reimbursement to medical providers that HEW (not the states) would design. Section

1902 a 13 B required that states provide for "payment of the reasonable cost (as determined in accordance with standards approved by the Secretary and included in the plan) of inpatient hospital services provided under the plan" (SSA 1965). Using *reasonable cost* as the basis of reimbursement for providers created strong inflationary incentives and contributed profoundly to the rapid and persistent rise in state medicaid expenditures during the late 1960s and 1970s.[7]

Joining the medicaid program and accepting these conditions-of-aid was in theory optional for states. Yet the fiscal and political pressures to extend public health care induced all but two states (Arizona and Alaska) to join by the 1970 deadline for the termination of Kerr-Mills. Despite the complexity and requirements of the program, five states enrolled by the end of 1966; and 32 more joined them by the end of 1968 (Thompson 1981, 117).

In 1967, very shortly after the initial enactment, Congress imposed further requirements upon the states—that they establish an Early and Periodic Screening, Diagnosis and Treatment Program, designed to seek eligible children to test and treat. Thompson reports that this policy was adopted by Congress without much "scrutiny of its potential costs or administrative problems"(1981, 122).

The medicaid legislation of 1965 and expansions enacted immediately thereafter illustrate the rising assertiveness of the federal government in intergovernmental relations. In the 1970s Congress retreated somewhat by loosening the provisions that states must expand their programs and must use *reasonable cost* as the basis for provider reimbursement. Some of the earlier permissiveness returned, but the foundation for the mandates of the 1980s had been laid.

CONCLUSION

The increase in medicaid spending in the late 1980s depended on congressional mandates. A series of mandatory expansions in eligibility and benefits, and the numerous other costly requirements that Congress imposed upon the states, represented an unusual degree of coerciveness in federal state relations. It is unlikely that these mandates would have been enacted, or would have been as intrusive, had a major change in federal-state relations not already been well underway. At least since the 1950s, the norms of federalism had been undergoing a prolonged transformation in which the federal government had become more assertive. Medicaid from its founding had exemplified the new pattern, albeit with some lingering ambiguity and inconsistency. Without this broad undercurrent of institutional change, the medicaid expansions of the 1980s would have been unthinkable.

NOTES

1. Only Governor Cuomo (D-NY), a notable liberal governor representing a state with one of the most generous medicaid programs, did not support this measure.

2. Hart instructs that prohibited actions include: "abusive actions by states legislatures and administrative officers"(1955, 196). Other prohibitions are specifically outlined in the Constitution itself, which forbids states to "pass any Bill of Attainder, ex post facto Law, or Law Impairing the Obligation of Contracts."

3. However, even this early measure included a surprisingly burdensome requirement that instructed states to provide for *the establishment or designation of a State authority or authorities which shall be responsible for establishing and maintaining standards* of care for patients in public or private health care institutions (SSA 1950, Title I, Section 2 A 9). This provision reappeared in each of its two successors.

4. The matching formula was based upon state per capita income, and ranged from 50 to 80 percent.

5. In 1962, Congress created two other categories to include the Blind and Permanently and Totally Disabled.

6. This had resulted in varying levels of program funding within the same state.

7. Although Congress granted states greater discretion in designing alternative payment systems in 1972, administrative obstacles still existed to their ability to use other methods. Not until 1980 and 1981 did the Boren Amendments offer the states additional leeway in establishing more efficient payment systems.

CHAPTER SIX

Changes in Institutions: The Budget Process

Bringing medicaid expansion to the congressional agenda was the easy part. Consideration of medicaid enlargements reached the floor of at least one chamber in 1977, 1978, and 1980. At that time the proposal enjoyed broad appeal among interest groups, Congress, and the president. Yet, despite the presence of Democratic majorities in both chambers, opponents, including fiscal conservatives and anti-abortion activists, were able to derail its passage. Getting medicaid extension to the congressional agenda was no assurance of its enactment.

The obstacles to such enactment—the opposition of the president, a divided government, and the existence of persistent and serious fiscal constraints—were even greater in the 1980s than earlier. How did advocates overcome these barriers to medicaid's adoption, not just once, but repeatedly between 1984 and 1990? The answer, quite simply, was that during the 1980s the congressional budget process changed. In both formal and informal ways Congress altered the process so that it created a unique vehicle for speeding measures through, allowing little opportunity for debate, opposition, alteration, or veto. Medicaid advocates in Congress recognized the opportunity this process provided and they exploited it. In nearly every year between 1984 and 1990, they linked their proposal for expansion to this bill. Doing so guaranteed medicaid a place on the annual agenda, limited the impact of opposition through minimizing debate, and permitted advocates to hide the full cost of enlargements. Without the unique advantages of this vehicle, the scope of medicaid extensions would certainly have been much smaller.

Congress is forever tinkering with its budget process, and in 1990 members again changed it in such a way as to create new obstacles to program expansions. And, not coincidentally, the extensions in medicaid then halted abruptly. This was not because the problems of health care coverage had been resolved; nor was it because the issue of access to health care dropped from the political agenda. Although health insurance for poor children improved during the late 1980s, the total number of uninsured continued to increase (Levit et al. 1992, 35). The election of Democratic underdog Harris Wofford to the Senate from Pennsylvania in 1991, based largely upon his promise of access to health care, and the priority that Bill Clinton placed on improving access to health care in his presidential campaign in 1992, demonstrate the enduring relevance of the issue after 1990. Although the House Energy and Commerce Committee continued to support the extension of medicaid in the early 1990s, it was unable to win any significant enlargements. Critical changes in the budget process, enacted as part of the 1990 Budget Enforcement Act, derailed the annual "express train" that medicaid advocates relied upon for expansions.

Two important changes in the congressional budget process promoted medicaid's adoption. First, during the early 1980s, Congress began employing the previously ignored mechanism created by the 1974 Budget Act, the *reconciliation process*, in order to facilitate changes in entitlement programs. Designed to provide Congress a mechanism for cutting back entitlement spending to conform to revenues, *reconciliation* contained special rules for limiting debate and facilitating consideration of such controversial measures. Reagan first recognized and exploited this process in 1981 to enact deep cut backs in entitlements. Then, later in the decade, the Democratic-controlled Congress turned the intended purpose of this process on its head. Instead of enacting reductions in entitlements, it found this process to be an excellent mechanism for enlarging the medicaid program.

A second important change in the budget process that aided in medicaid's adoption during the 1980s was enactment of the Balanced Budget and Emergency Deficit Control Act of 1985 (Gramm-Rudman-Hollings or GRH). Frustrated by its inability to reduce spending, Congress adopted GRH. Framed by Senators Phil Gramm (R-TX), Warren Rudman (R-NH), and Ernest F. Hollings (D-SC), this measure established a process designed to permit Congress to impose discipline upon itself to reduce the deficit. It set a goal to balance the budget within five years by establishing annual deficit targets and an enforcement mechanism to make certain Congress adhered to them. If the budget deficit was projected to exceed the target, and Congress and the White House could not agree on cuts or spending increases that year, then automatic cuts—sequestration—would be invoked. "Sequestration was the core concept of GRH," according to Davidson and Oleszek (1994, 401). However, medicaid was exempted from the sequestration, thus allowing members to enlarge that program without invoking sequestration. Another important way in which GRH facilitated the adoption of enlargements in medicaid was through permitting advocates to engage in accounting gimmicks that hid the full cost of medicaid changes (Schick 1995). GRH contained a number of flaws that made it a weak instrument of budget control, but one of its most serious was its lack of long-term budgeting requirements. By demanding only one-year budget targets, advocates had no difficulty in expanding medicaid while hiding the future costs of the program.

RECONCILIATION

Limited Debate

Reconciliation is a must-pass omnibus legislative vehicle that limits consideration, debate and opposition, including a presidential veto. In an attempt to reign in the growth of entitlements in 1980, Congress employed the long-ignored *reconciliation* process. It altered the budget process by moving *reconciliation* to the beginning of the budget calendar year, abandoning the use of the second resolution, and instructing authorizing committees to report changes in spending that conformed to the first budget resolution. This greatly increased the importance of *reconciliation* as a means of controlling entitlement spending.

Reconciliation contains two stages: issuing *reconciliation instructions* and enacting a *reconciliation bill. Reconciliation instructions* are a set of directions to designated committees[1] to report legislation by a certain deadline that will decrease entitlement spending or increase revenues by a designated amount. These *instructions* are contained in the budget *resolution*, which establishes budget targets for each functional area of the budget. The budget resolution is a very important document, setting the congressional budget priorities, and although the President does not sign it, this measure must be adopted in identical form by both chambers of Congress.[2]

In the *resolution*, the budget committees in each chamber issue separate *instructions* to their respective authorizing committees. These *instructions* are often accompanied by a report which outlines the assumptions regarding specific programs. Although the *instructions* are binding, the assumptions are not; committees possess much discretion regarding how they arrive at their assigned target figures. The authorizing committees submit their individual reconciliation proposals to the budget committees, which then compile them into the omnibus reconciliation bill without making any substantive changes. The entire reconciliation bill is then sent to the floor under certain rules for passage (Gilmour 1990, 95-98). In recent years, these bills have grown to great lengths.

Schick reports that, "the initial use of *reconciliation* was quite limited. Outlay savings were limited to a single fiscal year and totaled only about $4 billion" (1990, 90). However, its advantages as a legislative "express train" zooming through Congress soon became apparent (Gilmour 1990, 159). During a period of divided government, fiscal constraints, and anti-government sentiment among the public, reconciliation came to be recognized as a powerful legislative vehicle for the party that could control it. It promoted the adoption of measures that members managed to pack into it, which were less likely to be authorized if considered alone.

In 1981, with a Republican Senate and an ideologically split Democratic party exerting little control over the House, the Republicans were able to build consensus among fiscal conservatives to control the process. Recognizing the advantages of limiting debate and amendments, Reagan used the reconciliation process to help promote the adoption of sweeping budget cuts in domestic programs, including medicaid. Under continued fiscal pressures during the 1980s, Congress adopted some form of reconciliation measure every year. But, because of partisan changes, the Republicans were not able to gain control of the process again during that decade.

Increased Democratic party influence in the House and greater party unity during the 1980s played a significant role in permitting the Democratic party to control the terms of debate for consideration of the budget (Palazzo 1992, 122). Because of their unusual advantages, reconciliation bills have become one of the most popular mechanisms in Congress for attaching unrelated riders that might not otherwise be adopted (Rovner, 1989, 964).

Representative Pete Stark (D-CA), chair of the House Ways and Means Committee's Subcommittee on Health said, "The Stark Strategy is if we can see an opening, we'll go for it and take whatever little pieces of legislation we can get and sneak them in reconciliation" (quoted in Rovner 1989, 966). The importance of reconciliation is echoed by Representative Bill Gradison (R-OH), ranking member of the same subcommittee. He said, "I like reconciliation. It gives us a chance to do things we otherwise couldn't do" (quoted in Rovner 1989, 966). The enlargement of the medicaid program was one of the things included in nearly every reconciliation bill between 1984 and 1990 that might not otherwise have been possible.

Reconciliation helped medicaid expansions by ensuring that they would be included in the "must-pass" omnibus measures, which were considered under limited debate and protected from amendments and presidential vetoes.[3] Packaging them in such large bills protected them from the scrutiny and vulnerability of proposals that are considered alone. Diane Rowland, Executive Director of the Kaiser Commission on the Future of Medicaid and legislative aide to Rep. Henry Waxman during the 1980s, remarked, "If [the medicaid enlargements] had not been part of the reconciliation bill, none of this could have happened." She continued, "Reconciliation is a vehicle that is hard to amend" (Interview 1992).

Omnibus reconciliation bills limit debate in part by overwhelming legislators with their sheer size. Since so many issues are considered simultaneously in an omnibus bill, members of Congress have little time (or inclination) to learn the specifics, especially if the issue produces no major controversy (Fuchs and Hoadley 1987, 218). Advocates for medicaid's enlargement were fortunate in this respect. No well-organized and direct opposition emerged among interest groups. Fiscal conservatives including President Bush were often supportive of medicaid expansions, although of a much smaller magnitude than those proposed by liberal Democrats.

Because of their size, reconciliation bills provide effective cover to legislators who wish to avoid being held accountable by their constituents for an unpopular vote. Such strategies have become increasingly popular according to Arnold (1990, 102). During an era of large deficits, the public and members of Congress are torn between their desire for continuation of their favorite government programs and deficit reduction (Davidson and Olezek 1994, 405).

Wildavsky explains that, "Deficit panic is an elite phenomenon," suggesting that most of the public are not greatly concerned about the deficit (1992, 219). Legislators, nevertheless, fear being accused of irresponsible spending. Arnold argues that legislators must take into consideration not only the actual effects of legislation they support, but,

> At the same time, the potential for policy voting forces them to consider how their positions on various issues will sound to citizens . . . Issues related to welfare also raise problems for many legislators, given the popular image of those who accept such assistance (1990, 78-80).

Omnibus legislation provides cover for those legislators for whom expanding the deficit, especially for an unpopular clientele such as the poor, may present a problem back home. Inserting medicaid enlargement in the reconciliation bill reduced opposition and discouraged amendments.

Another way that reconciliation protected medicaid was through offering an unusual degree of protection from presidential vetoes. Because of the ideological differences between congressional Democrats and President Reagan, the use of omnibus measures increased during the 1980s in order to avoid possible vetoes (Sinclair 1989, 35). Although the adoption of reconciliation legislation is not required, because of the importance of budget deficit legislation, Congress has enacted such legislation for each fiscal year during the 1980s. And despite threats to the contrary, the president signed each of them. Reagan was opposed to medicaid extensions, and he repeatedly threatened to veto the budget bill if they were included; however, because of the urgency of deficit control, he could not afford to follow through (Congressional Quarterly Almanac, hereafter CQA 1987, 626). Without such protection, his veto was assured. Richard Kogan, legislative staff member of the House Budget Committee during the 1980s, acknowledged that reconciliation offered "the only chance to get medicaid expansions without a Reagan veto" (Interview 1995). In 1989 and again in 1990, Bush also threatened to veto the budget bill because of medicaid enlargements that exceeded his more modest proposals.

His threat was taken seriously, and may have kept advocates in Congress from pushing for even greater extensions.

Perhaps the most important way in which reconciliation minimized debate and muted opposition to medicaid enlargements was through the use of restrictive rules for considering that measure. Both chambers limit debate for considering the budget resolution and reconciliation bill; however, the rules and norms for considering the budget in the House are under greater control of the leadership of the majority party. Because of the majority status of the Democratic party in that chamber during the 1980s, the Democratic leadership had much influence over the budget process. Majorities in the authorizing committees assured that the Democratic agenda would be proposed. Furthermore, because of the role that both the Budget and Rules Committees played as tools of the leadership,[4] these committees helped assure that the agenda of the Democratic party would be promoted through the budget process. The Budget Committee made certain that the instructions given the authorizing committee would include funds for their programs; and the Rules Committee would deliver a restricted rule that precluded debate for the measures supported by the leadership.

Given the structure of the budget process, once authorizing committees include a proposal in the reconciliation bill, little opportunity exists to change it. The budget committee is not allowed to make substantive alteration, and the restriction on amendments from the floor further heightens the influence of the authorizing committees. According to Fuchs and Hoadley, "Members not on the major health committees have very few opportunities to have any input . . . This concentration of policymaking power substantially narrows the circle of involved actors" (1987, 218). The House Energy and Commerce Committee (HECC), with strong Democratic advocates of medicaid expansion, possesses sole jurisdiction over that program in the House. And, although partisan control of the budget process was not as strong in the Senate, the Finance Committee had exclusive jurisdiction over medicaid in that chamber.

Because the Democratic leaders in the House were committed to a liberal agenda that included expanding social welfare programs for the poor, and they possessed the capacity to limit amending activity in that chamber, they took advantage of the opportunity. Steven Smith documents the increase in restrictive rules during the 1980s (Smith 1989, 339). One motivation for this, according to Smith, is the

"Democrats shared a collective party interest in reducing the policy and political damage of Republican amendments . . . the move to more restrictive rules was reinforced by budget dominated politics of the 1980s" (339-340). Not surprisingly, the result has been to produce greater party-line voting on the budget (Davidson and Olezek 1994, 405). Democrats in the House included medicaid enlargement in nearly every reconciliation measure between 1984 and 1990; and they adopted a restricted rule for every single reconciliation bill considered during the decade.

Numerical majorities and a high level of party unity on budget-related matters during the 1980s easily enabled the Democrats on the authorizing committee to limit opposition and amendments at that level. The minority party attempted to reduce or eliminate an increase in medicaid from the agenda on several occasions within the HECC and its Subcommittee on Health, but they failed each time.

In the debate surrounding the 1986 FY budget, for example, the Republicans on the HECC objected to extensions in medicaid, but by a vote of 22-6, were unable to prevent the committee from passing them. James T. Broyhill (R-NC) argued, "I don't want to argue the merits of these spending proposals . . . But it's totally inappropriate to consider them as part of the [budget] reconciliation process" (Hook 1985, 1554). He recognized and objected to the exploitation of the budget process by Democrats but was powerless to stop them.

Again, in 1987, Republicans on the HECC proved unable to block enlargements in medicaid. An amendment by Rep. William E. Dannemeyer (R-CA) to remove all health provisions that increased spending was defeated 5-14. And by a vote of 22-4, the panel adopted health care expansions, including those in medicaid, that the CBO estimated would cost nearly $500 million over three years.

In 1989, Rep. Edward Madigan (R-IL) offered an amendment supported by President Bush that would have provided less generous coverage to near-poor pregnant women and infants than what the Democrats on the HECC Subcommittee on Health had proposed. This measure failed on a 7-11 party-line vote. The full committee finally adopted sizable expansions in the medicaid program by a 29-14 vote with three Republican defectors. These examples illustrate the limited opportunity at the committee-level for changing medicaid legislation under reconciliation.

Democratic control over the Rules Committee also muted Republican objections and attempts to derail extensions in medicaid. Republicans frequently opposed the rule because of fiscal concerns. One year in particular stimulated vocal complaints. In considering the rule for the 1986 FY reconciliation bill, shortly after Congress adopted the GRH bill for deficit reduction, Republicans proposed five separate amendments, each of which was defeated on a party-line vote. One such amendment, proposed by Rep. Willis D. Gradison (R-OH), would have eliminated all new spending from the reconciliation bill. The Rules panel finally proposed a closed rule. Not one Republican voted for it. Limiting amendments when considering medicaid was another important advantage the budget process offered medicaid advocates because of opposition from those members who wished to reshape the medicaid program in other ways. "With an ordinary bill," one House Democratic aide acknowledged, "we don't have the votes on the floor to protect us from abortion amendments or nasty AIDS amendments" (Rovner 1989, 968).

Reconciliation presented the Democratic leadership in the House the opportunity to control the terms of debate and promote the adoption of medicaid expansions; this was not true, however, in the Senate. Leadership in the Senate is different from the House. The Senate lacks the strong rules and procedures of the House, as its norms promote more bipartisan discussion (Davidson, 1989, 292). Furthermore, the amendment process in the Senate is less structured, generally relying upon agreements reached by party leaders through broad consultation (Schick 1995, 75).

The Senate standing rules, rather than the decision of a specific committee, limit debate of the reconciliation measure to 20 hours, precluding filibuster or other delaying tactics. This restricts consideration of the entire bill to 12 minutes per member, or "barely one minute per page," in some years, according to Schick (1995, 85). These rules support the Senate's conventional responsibility as guardian of the purse. Schick explains,

> The rules in the House are designed to facilitate the passage of legislation produced by committees. The Senate's are designed to constrain the spending ambitions of committees and members (1995, 95).

This more open process of debate, along with the Senate's traditional role of considering the President's requests[5] (Davidson 1989, 297), and the more fiscally conservative nature of Senators of both parties, meant that the Senate in the 1980s was less inclined than the House to support expansions in social welfare program, such as medicaid.

Increased Importance of Conference Negotiations

Given how far apart the House and Senate were on the issue of medicaid enlargements, reconciliation was an important mechanism for ensuring that it reached the conference. This process assures that authorization bills will be included in conference even if they are opposed by the other chamber (Davidson 1992, 263). When Congress considers an omnibus measure, if one chamber rejects the bill, it does not die. If one chamber rejects part of the bill, it will still be considered in conference. This feature of omnibus bills minimizes the need for advocates to win broad support in both chambers and enhances the significance of conference negotiations.

Important differences emerged between the House and the Senate positions on medicaid increases. Part of the explanation resides in the different institutional roles of the two chambers as discussed above. Another reason is partisan politics. Republicans controlled the Senate for the first three years of this study, and enlargement of social programs was not one of their priorities. Even when the Democrats controlled the Senate in the late 1980s, they were ideologically split with more fiscally conservative members than in the House. These Senators were less likely to support an increase in medicaid or support it as fully under intense fiscal pressures. Consequently, the Senate was less consistent and less generous in its proposals to expand the medicaid program between the years 1984 and 1990. (See Table 6.1 for a summary of those differences.)

The size of conference negotiations also worked to the advantage of medicaid. Because of the size and complexity of the reconciliation bills during the 1980s, the conference committees considering them were also unusually large. Conference committees were broken into subconferences so as to expedite the work. Decisionmaking was structured in such a way that only the few conferees within a particular

Table 6.1: Senate Position on Budget Reconciliation

Budget for Fiscal Year	Senate Position on Medicaid Expansions at Time of Conference Committee
1985	Less generous expansion than House
1986	Sought cuts, no expansions
1987	Strong bipartisan support for expansions
1988	Strong bipartisan opposition to expansions after Stock Market crash
1989	Not included in budget legislation
1990	No true expansion beyond inflation
1991	Less generous expansion than House

subconference would vote upon that portion of the omnibus measure. This feature of the conference committee limited the opportunity for opposition and allowed negotiators in subconference to exert great influence over the final shape of the legislation. After conferees signed off on their subconference agreement, each chamber received only one opportunity to vote up or down on the entire package.

The leadership of each chamber decided who would be assigned to the subconferences; and appointments were made according to various criteria, including seniority and interest in the legislation. In each case, Henry Waxman, as chair of the Subcommittee on Health and the Environment that recommended medicaid enlargement, and a powerful advocate, was assigned to the subconference on medicaid.

When monetary differences between the House and Senate versions of a bill arise, as they did for enlargements in medicaid in 1984 and 1990, the conferees often average the difference between the two figures (Oleszek 1996, 285). In both cases, the initial House figure was significantly reduced in conference. However, if one chamber rejects additions outright, as the Senate did in 1986, 1987, and 1989, compromise is more complex. Oleszek suggests logrolling may result, "with House conferees agreeing to certain Senate-passed provisions to gain leverage to win acceptance of House-passed provisions elsewhere in the bill that are strongly supported by members of their own chamber offers and counter offers are part of the often exhausting conference process" (Olezek 1996, 285). This sort of negotiating characterized the budget conferences of the late 1980s, according to one Democratic aide to the HECC. Such complex negotiations require not only multiple actors, but the skill of the negotiators assumes great importance (Oleszek 1996, 286).

The structure of conference committees for reconciliation bills assured that each year during the 1980s, even if the Senate voted to oppose any medicaid extension, its conferees would be forced to negotiate in subconference with a House conferee who chaired the subcommittee advocating annual expansions in that program, Henry Waxman (D-CA). And Waxman is a formidable negotiator. Thus, differences between the two chambers on medicaid meant that Senate conferees would face tough negotiations with the House, and, given the importance of medicaid extensions to the House leadership, logrolling would not result in the House abandoning this measure. The Senate would then be unlikely to avoid including some level of medicaid enlargement in the final version of the reconciliation bill.

The *reconciliation* process lent itself to incremental additions in medicaid. Even if advocates failed to win large increases in conference in any particular year, they were assured of being able to try again the next year. Through using the process year after year, they accumulated a series of changes, sometimes relatively small ones, that amounted to a major extension in medicaid benefits and eligibility over the course of the decade.

GRAMM-RUDMAN-HOLLINGS

In addition to reconciliation, the adoption of the Balanced Budget and Emergency Deficit Control Act of 1985 (Gramm-Rudman-Hollings or GRH) promoted medicaid enlargement in two important ways: by promoting the choice of medicaid over other alternatives and by permitting advocates to hide its long term costs.

The process contained serious flaws as a means of decreasing the deficit, and did not live up to its expectations. Some have argued GRH promoted larger budgets than earlier (Ferejohn 1991; Ferejohn and Krehbiel 1987). Others are more specific, suggesting that certain programs were advantaged by GRH—namely those, such as medicaid, that were exempt from sequestration (Hahm et al. 1992):

> Programs exempt from sequester have no incentive to contribute budgetary reductions in order to accommodate a budget package that avoids sequestration . . . GRH appears to have restrained outlays for

non-exempt programs below levels that would have prevailed in the absence of GRH. No such restraining effect for programs exempt from sequestration is observed. If anything, these programs experienced a modest expansionary impact from GRH (1992, 212-213, 222).

This research indicates that exemption from sequestration provided a "modest" stimulus toward program expansion. By setting deficit targets and establishing an enforcement mechanism while exempting medicaid, GRH made it relatively easier for Congress to choose medicaid for enlargements over other non-exempt programs.[6]

This situation eliminated a number of policy options from consideration and highlighted the fiscal advantages of medicaid's shared funding with the states. The threat of sequestration made shared funding even more significant, since Congress could derive political benefits from expanding such a program at only half the cost. Other fully federally funded programs did not enjoy this advantage. In fact, under the tight fiscal circumstances of the 1980s, being fully federally funded not only hindered the chances of enlarging other health care programs, but made them more attractive to budget cutters. Rovner describes how GRH increased the importance of program funding. She explains that a disproportionate amount of medicare cutbacks have come from Part A rather than Part B, because, "only three-quarters of Part B is financed by the federal government (the remainder comes from premiums), so each dollar cut only 'scores' as 75 cents saved" (1989, 968). Because they are fully federally funded, discretionary programs and medicare (Part A) suffered serious cutbacks during the mid- and late-1980s, while medicaid did not attract such attention.

The second important way that GRH promoted the enlargement of medicaid was through hiding its long term costs. Although reconciliation permitted Congress to establish either single- or multiple-year budgets, in some years Congress chose the latter. This option minimized the ability of members to use accounting gimmicks to achieve savings.[7] In 1981 *reconciliation* was stretched to three years, "to spur committees to produce permanent savings" (Schick 1990, 91). However, with a change in partisan influence and agendas in 1984, Congress opted to employ single year budget reconciliation bills for the rest of the decade. GRH permitted, and even encouraged, single year accountability. It only required that the cost of increases that applied to the current year be used to determine whether a change in a program met the deficit target. This opened the door to accounting gimmicks that shifted the cost to future years. Thus, Congress could claim to be fulfilling the letter of the law, while avoiding the reality of having increased expenditures. According to Schick,

> GRH started out as a process for reducing the deficit and has become a means of hiding the deficit and running away from responsibility for. . . . it gives politicians a strong incentive to schedule increased spending in the current rather than the next year's budget . . . In fact, [GRH] puts a premium on one-year-at-a-time behavior. All that matters is the single year for which projections are being made (1990, 205).

By permitting advocates to hide the full cost of medicaid's expansions, GRH helped promote the adoption of that policy. Joseph White refers to the use of reconciliation to hide such changes in the medicaid program as the "epitome of an inside game" (1996, 60). Congressional advocates for medicaid adhered to the technical requirements of GRH while accruing large, long-term costs. Support for the extension of medicaid was enhanced in 1989 and again in 1990 through altering the beginning date of the measure until late in the fiscal year. "We called these the budgetary time bombs," according to Dan Gengler from OMB (Morgan 1994a). Others referred to them as "the Waxman wedge," because of the role that subcommittee chair played in orchestrating this strategy. A former CBO official Dan Muse stated, "[Waxman staffers] would have us move the [effective date of the legislation], or the ages of the eligible beneficiaries, until they got what they needed. Waxman had a pot of money, and he would make the totals match what was in the budget resolution" (Morgan 1994a). GRH allowed this sort of gimmickry, and medicaid advocates exploited it.

BUDGET ENFORCEMENT ACT OF 1990

Because of the inadequacies of GRH, Congress again officially altered the budget process in 1990 through enacting the Budget Enforcement Act (BEA). This legislation erected significant barriers to further adoption of medicaid enlargements. With the passage of the 1990 BEA,

Diane Rowland remarked, "The window that was opened, not very wide, closed" (Interview 1992). Establishing a three-year budget removed the annual reconciliation bill and its one-year targets from the agenda, forcing advocates of program expansions to be explicit about the long-term costs of such program changes.

One of the most important aspects of the BEA was PAYGO, the requirement that no program extensions would be allowed unless they were accompanied by commensurate adjustments in revenues or cuts in other programs. This prerequisite erected "a parliamentary stumbling block for issues once they reached the floor" according to Senate Budget Committee aide, Kathy Deignan (Interview 1995). Richard Kogan explains that PAYGO "segmented the world into discretionary and entitlement spending." Advocates of medicaid or medicare could not squeeze appropriations to pay for expansions in those programs. As a result, he claims, "competition became fiercer." Furthermore, he reports that after 1990 "the House Ways and Means Committee adopted the attitude that they wouldn't cut medicare for medicaid, but only for the overall deficit" (Interview 1995). The new requirements and the unwillingness of HWMC to cooperate created powerful obstacles to increases in medicaid.

The 1984-1990 enlargements in medicaid had been strongly dependent upon omnibus reconciliation measures as the legislative vehicle. However, another change in the budget process made the annual reconciliation bill unnecessary. A three-year budget agreement was established as part of the OBRA of 1990 (Feder and Rowland 1992, 362). This had two serious consequences for advocates of medicaid extensions. It meant budget figures were binding for three years, rather than merely one. Such a requirement made the long term cost of medicaid extensions explicit. Richard Kogan reports this change "minimized the possibility of gaming the system" (Interview 1995). Members of Congress would have to make a choice to support extensions in medicaid knowing the full cost of such a change. In addition, the three year budget agreement adopted as part of the BEA removed the need for an annual reconciliation bill. Consequently, Congress did not enact a reconciliation bill in 1991 or 1992. Given the obstacles erected by BEA, advocates have been unsuccessful in gaining any significant medicaid enlargements since 1990.

CONCLUSION

Although a positive political atmosphere promoting the enlargement of medicaid emerged in the 1980s, the adoption of that policy was by no means guaranteed. Important institutional developments, including changes in the congressional budget process, gave advocates an important legislative vehicle for overcoming the numerous obstacles to medicaid enlargement that existed during the 1980s—the opposition of the President, a divided government, and the existence of persistent and serious fiscal constraints. By linking proposals for medicaid expansion to the annual budget reconciliation bill, advocates enhanced the chances of their enactment. Reconciliation assured medicaid additions a place on the annual agenda, minimized debate, limited the impact of opposition from fiscal conservatives, and facilitated their adoption through permitting advocates to hide the full cost of such a policy. Both before 1984 and after 1990 obstacles to the enactment of medicaid extensions proved insurmountable. Without the advantages of the reconciliation budget process of the 1980s, the succession of medicaid extensions enacted in that decade would not have been possible. Whereas the budget reconciliation process provided advocates the opportunity for pushing the issue of medicaid expansion through Congress, the enactment of such a policy depended heavily upon their ability to take advantage of that opportunity. Without the political skill and determination of a powerful and strategically situated policy entrepreneur, the budget process might have gone untapped as a political tool. And, despite the political support for medicaid enlargements, they might have been either smaller in scale or nonexistent.

NOTES

1. Congress does not initiate *reconciliation* every year. It is an optional process that Congress can utilize to reduce the deficit or increase revenues. Such was the case during each year between 1980 and 1990. When multi-year budgets have been agreed to, reconciliation is less likely. Although reconciliation instructions might be used for any committee, Congress has only issued such instructions to committees with jurisdiction over revenues or mandatory spending programs (Schick 1995, 82-83).

2. The House considers the *budget resolution* under a limited rule; and the Senate rules only permit 50 hours of debate.

3. Although reconciliation was not intended to serve as a vehicle for program expansions, medicaid's entitlement status meant that any change in it—including expansion—is considered germane (Fuchs and Hoadley 1987, 217).

4. The Rules Committee was dominated by Democrats loyal to the Speaker by virtue of having been appointed by him (Dodd and Oppenheimer 1989, 52). Sinclair claims that the party leadership decides what new programs may be included in the reconciliation bill that carries out the budget resolution (1989, 315).

5. President Reagan was opposed to medicaid expansions and President Bush only supported those that were inflation neutral.

6. According to Hahm et al., medicaid is the only health care program that was fully exempt from GRH sequestration. Medicare was partially protected. It could be reduced under sequestration only 1 or 2 percent, depending upon the year (1992, 218-219).

7. In 1980 some committees met their target figures by temporary savings or through manipulating the starting date of certain payments (Schick 1990, 90-91).

CHAPTER SEVEN

The Role of the Policy Entrepreneur

While political and institutional changes were necessary conditions for medicaid's repeated enlargements, they were not sufficient. Without the skill and will of a powerful policy entrepreneur to take advantage of those unique circumstances, the sweeping extension of medicaid that occurred in the mid- to late-1980s would not have been possible. Henry A. Waxman (D-CA) is universally recognized among policy analysts as that person. He was the prime mover in exploiting those circumstances to establish medicaid expansion on the congressional agenda, to ensure it remained there, and to help push for the adoption of the greatest possible extension by Congress.

Policy entrepreneurs have long been important to greasing the wheels of Congress and promoting passage of legislation. A study conducted by John Kingdon in the early 1980s concluded that in 15 out of 23 case studies an entrepreneur was "very" or "somewhat important" in getting an item on the agenda (1984, 189). Such individuals are characterized by a "willingness to invest their resources—time, energy, reputation, and sometimes money—in the hope of a future return," according to Kingdon (1984, 129). Waxman exemplified these characteristics in pursuing passage of the medicaid program. Because of this pattern of behavior throughout his career, not only in regard to medicaid, he is viewed by some scholars as the premier example of a policy entrepreneur (Loomis 1989; Rhode 1991). Given the many obstacles to program enlargement that existed in the mid-1980s, such a role was even more critical.

Kingdon discusses the three types of benefits that motivate entrepreneurs: first, direct, personal or concrete rewards, such as re-election; second, an ability to promote their values and shape public policy; and third, enjoyment from being part of the action (Kingdon 1984, 129-30). Of these three benefits Waxman, who holds a relatively safe seat,[1] is arguably motivated most highly by a desire to shape policy. His choice to serve on the Energy and Commerce Committee is consistent with this goal. That panel is widely regarded as a policy committee, in contrast to others which primarily serve constituency or heighten influence and prestige (Smith and Deering 1990, 87). The House Energy and Commerce Committee "is on the cutting edge of fundamental issues that are central to the U.S. economy" (Plattner 1983, 501).

Waxman's motivation for pursuing health care and other social issues derives from his personal convictions. He was born in 1939, in the aftermath of the Depression, and was raised above his father's grocery store in south-central Los Angeles. After giving up the store, his father went to work for a large grocery chain and became active in the local retail clerks' union. These experiences helped to shape Waxman's values. He says, "My parents were very much affected by the way they viewed the world as a result of the Depression, and they revered Franklin Roosevelt." His father instilled the belief that "unless government plays a role in helping people who would otherwise be powerless, these people would easily be forgotten" (Morgan 1994a).

Some hold that his religious beliefs also play a large role in his policy positions. His grandparents were Russian Jewish immigrants who fled the pogroms of Europe. And Waxman fervently holds to the tenets of his Jewish faith—keeping Kosher, refusing to work on Saturday, and participating in his temple. He has said, "I think from a Jewish religious point of view, people have responsibility for others to try to bring about social justice and take care of people who can't take care of themselves" (Kosterlitz 1989, 577). This helps explain his commitment to the medicaid program.

Waxman's desire to shape policy does not mean that he does not also seek power and influence—for the evidence suggests otherwise. Such qualities are critical to one's ability to pursue policy goals.

QUALITIES OF AN ENTREPRENEUR

Kingdon describes three essential attributes of policy entrepreneurs (1984, 189-190). First, one must possess some claim to a hearing through expertise or by virtue of one's position of authoritative decision-making. Waxman demonstrated both of these; he is widely respected for his expertise on health care issues and he held the chair of a powerful subcommittee throughout the 1980s. During his tenure in the California Assembly, he first revealed his interest in health care policy. He has said, "I made a decision that I should specialize . . . if I were to have the opportunity to make an impact." He chose health policy because, according to Waxman, "I thought that there was a clear role for government to play that was unambiguous to most people" (Kosterlitz 1989, 578).

Furthermore, his position as chair of the Subcommittee on Health and the Environment of the HECC with jurisdiction over two major health care programs—medicare, part B and medicaid—also provides him with a claim to a hearing. It is "one of the half dozen most important subcommittees in the House," according to Barone and Ujifusa (1986, 154).

Second, Kingdon suggests an entrepreneur must be known for his negotiating skill or political connections. Waxman excels in these as well. His personality, described as "low-key, affable and modest," lends itself to working well with people. However, as one of his aides said, "It is not a fruit-and-nuts-California mellowness" (Kosterlitz 1989, 578). He was one of the first junior members of Congress to successfully challenge a more senior member for an important chairmanship. In order to assume the chair of the Subcommittee on Health and the Environment of the HECC in 1979, Waxman challenged and beat Richardson Preyer (D-NC), a respected member with greater seniority and who also had the support of the Democratic leadership, (Barone et al. 1980, 99-100).

Serving in that position heightens Waxman's political connections. The broad legislative jurisdiction of the HECC offered him great influence in the House, in part, because the committee controls so much spending (*CQA* 1986, 33). Serving on it provides members the opportunity to bargain with other legislators to obtain their votes on key issues. His chairmanship also provided Waxman access to significant amounts of PAC money. This money, along with that which he successfully solicited from his wealthy, liberal constituents for his own PAC and re-election campaign, enabled Waxman to contribute significant sums to the re-election of his colleagues, which he did— liberally.

From 1983 to 1989 Waxman contributed $558,000 to Democratic candidates' and members' campaigns. Kosterlitz reports that about one-fourth of that went to members of the HECC, and about two-thirds to his own sub-committee members. Between 1988 and 1990 Waxman "funneled more than $1 million to influential Democrats in the House and Senate. At the end of 1988, Waxman could look around at meetings of the HECC and see six colleagues who had received $40,000 from his 'leadership PAC' just within the previous two years" (Morgan 1994a).

His influence extends even beyond Congress. During the last years of the 1980s, Waxman also contributed $28,000 to candidates for the California State Assembly, which had the task of redrawing the congressional districts after 1990 (Kosterlitz 1989, 578). This illustrates Waxman's foresight and willingness to use his influence to assure his political security.

Another source of Waxman's political connections derives from his membership on the Democratic Steering and Policy Committee. Since this body assigns members to committees, it is of tremendous importance. Waxman has used his position to help place allies in important positions, such as Howard L. Berman, (D-CA) on the Budget Committee (Kosterlitz 1989, 578).

Waxman's willingness to use his influence has won him both high praise and sharp criticism from his colleagues. Former Rep. Buddy MacKay (D-FL) said of Waxman, "He's a legislator's legislator. It's unusual to have a guy who understands the system as well and is also a very compassionate person" (Kosterlitz 1989, 577). His detractors, while acknowledging his skill, describe him differently. An ally, George Miller (D-CA), recounts when he joined the Budget Committee, "I thought Henry's first name was 'sunuvabitch.' Everybody who had to deal with [him] kept saying, 'Do you know what that sunuvabitch Waxman wants now?' (Kosterlitz 1989, 577).

His negotiating skill in conference committee is legendary. During the mid-1980s Robert Dole (R-KA), then-Majority Leader in the Senate, warned his colleagues not to amend a bill on the floor because it would mean facing Waxman in conference (Kosterlitz, 579). Waxman's skill in negotiating arises in part from Kingdon's third essential quality of an entrepreneur—persistence. This persistence paid off in negotiations in conference committees, and was especially important in when the Senate and House differed in their treatment of medicaid—nearly every year between 1984 and 1990. (See Table 6.1 for the summary of differences between House and Senate positions at the time of conference committee negotiations).

Dan Morgan illustrates Waxman's persistence through the following account:

> It was 7:30 in the morning on Oct. 16, 1990, and Rep. Henry A. Waxman (D-Calif.) had just spent the night in a windowless room in the Capitol haggling with senators over mind-numbing technicalities of the budget for Medicaid, the huge federal-state health care program for the poor, disabled and low-income elderly.
>
> Officials and aides were "hallucinating, green," recalled one of those present. But the short, balding chairman of the House Energy and Commerce Committee's subcommittee on health and environment looked as fresh and chipper as if he had slept in his bed in Bethesda (1994a).

Such maneuvering during conference committee was not uncommon for Henry Waxman. A former Republican staffer on the subcommittee is quoted as saying, "Henry was a bulldog on this [medicaid expansions]. He was in there for the long haul. He struck me as someone who would be happy spending his whole life protecting the health of moms and kids" (Morgan 1994a).

In 1989 Waxman wrote, "Incrementalism may not get much press, but it does work" (1217). That philosophy of persistence and relying upon incremental changes to reach one's goals has been his consistent strategy. Beginning in 1984 and continuing through 1990 he worked actively to bring the health care needs of the poor to the national agenda, to assure that medicaid expansion was the chosen policy vehicle, and to gain congressional approval. His willingness and ability to exert influence at so many stages of the policy process were essential to medicaid's growth.

AGENDA SETTING

An essential role of policy entrepreneurs, according to Kingdon, is "coupling" or bringing together the three "streams" of events and activities that flow along independently—problem, policy, and politics. He suggests that fleeting "policy windows" open up that permit passage of certain measures. Policy entrepreneurs must be able to link these streams at the appropriate time if they wish to be successful in bringing their proposal to government's agenda. The political, institutional, and environmental factors which cause a policy window to open are out of the control of the entrepreneur, argues Kingdon, but these individuals lie in wait for the opportunity to push their pet proposal. He writes that they

> hook solutions to problems, proposals to political momentum, and political events to policy problems. Without the entrepreneur, the linking of the streams may not take place. Good ideas lie fallow for lack of an advocate. Problems are unsolved for lack of a solution. Political events are not capitalized for lack of inventive and developed proposals (191).

In the case of medicaid expansion, Waxman played an important role as coupler. He was influential in shaping the health care problem as one of access to care for poor pregnant women and children. He promoted medicaid expansion as the preferred policy solution, and he helped to build a political coalition to support that alternative. He did not sit passively waiting for policy windows to open wide, but he persistently took advantage of the tiniest crack to nudge his proposal forward.

Problem

Problems of rising health care costs and decreasing access to care affected many groups in society during the 1980s. These difficulties were exacerbated for the poor after the OBRA cuts of 1981. Waxman skillfully shaped the issue to focus upon the problem for one particularly vulnerable segment of the population, and arguably the most severely affected, poor pregnant women and children. Waxman's choice to focus on poor children was good politics, strengthening support for his proposal. Furthermore, the plight of many poor children worsened as a result of the 1981 OBRA cuts, helping to lend legitimacy for government involvement in a problem it helped to create.

Kingdon says that persuasion is the main way in which an entrepreneur is able to succeed in defining a particular problem. Waxman helped to persuade his colleagues and the interested public that this problem deserved attention through generating information in support of his position and publicizing that perspective. He used three main mechanisms:

1. In 1983 and 1985 Waxman's subcommittee held hearings on medicaid and maternal-child health.

2. His subcommittee requested the congressional Office of Technology Assessment to conduct a study and publish a report on child health issues. It analyzed the cost-effectiveness of a policy of medicaid eligibility for all pregnant women with incomes below the federal poverty level and reached the conclusion that the expense of additional prenatal coverage would be highly cost-effective, in contrast to the expense of hospitalization and long term treatment of low-birthweight infants (Sardell 1991, 31-33).

3. He also advocated the creation of the House Select Committee on Children, Youth and Families in 1983. His friend and medicaid ally, Rep. George Miller (D-CA), was selected chair of that committee. This panel held hearings around the nation to help highlight children's health issues.

As the 1980s progressed, Waxman continued to promote the expansion of medicaid to provide access to health care for poor children. Then, as health care problems worsened for other poor and near-poor groups in society, he began to expand his focus to include them as well. Once the problem of access to care for the poor was viewed as a legitimate topic on the agenda, it was not difficult to expand the agenda to include other groups, such as unemployed families, the homeless, aliens, and the poor elderly.

Policy

It was perhaps natural for Waxman to push for an expansion of medicaid, the federal-state shared health care program for the poor, over which his committee had sole jurisdiction. However, it was not mere convenience that led Waxman to such a policy. Expanding that program met other criteria which Kingdon points out are critical for selection among alternatives.

One of the most important was fiscal constraints. While no one could accurately project the costs of the program extension, Waxman was quite skillful in manipulating the amount that appeared on the budget. Waxman's aides would write a proposal so it would begin late in the fiscal year, so the true fiscal impact would not be felt for a couple of years. Donald Muse, a former official at the Office of the Management of the Budget, claimed that Waxman's aides would manipulate several variables—say, the effective date of legislation or the age of eligibles—trying to get the first year estimates to equal the budgetary requirements (Morgan 1994a).

A long softening up process that allows members of Congress and the policy community to become familiar with a particular policy also helps promote its acceptance. Kingdon cites a political appointee who explains:

> A lot of preconditioning has to happen. This town does not respond instantaneously to a new idea. There has to be a lot of preconditioning, a lot of maneuvering in the first place (1984, 137).

Waxman certainly emulated this approach. He sponsored or supported medicaid expansions in the House for six of the seven years between 1977 and 1983[2] before they were finally enacted in 1984. His persistence paid off so that by 1984 medicaid extension was no longer a new idea.

Politics

Several political factors aided Waxman's efforts as the decade wore on. Worsening health care conditions helped promote the growth of a coalition supporting medicaid enlargement, and elections brought an increasingly liberal Congress. Sizable bipartisan support emerged in Congress as a result. In addition, a change in the administration aided Waxman's position; George Bush had campaigned on a platform of expanding medicaid in 1988.

The political philosophy of Reagan and Bush that promoted a *new federalism* also assisted Waxman in gaining support for a proposal that shifted responsibilities to the states. Ronald Reagan had capitalized upon this philosophy to decrease the federal commitment to medicaid and other social programs in the early 1980s. Waxman then exploited this view to expand both the federal and state commitments to medicaid in the mid 1980s. Permitting the states to expand medicaid through optional measures made this strategy difficult for Reagan supporters to oppose, according to Kosterlitz (1989, 580). Later measures involved less state discretion, but still allowed Waxman to utilize the rhetoric of shifting greater responsibility to the states.

Kingdon argues that, unlike in the *problem* and *policy streams*, coalitions in the *political stream* are built through bargaining rather than persuasion. Waxman possessed an ample supply of resources to utilize both strategies. He was aided somewhat by the evolving political mood and elections that were more favorable to medicaid expansion, and by the fact that no powerful opponents to helping poor children emerged.[3]

Therefore, Waxman was able to rely heavily upon what Davidson and Oleszek term *implicit bargaining* to build support in Congress. Waxman's position as chairman of the Subcommittee on Health and the Environment and his well-recognized expertise enabled him to enlist the backing of those members who lacked much interest or expertise on medicaid. Members could reasonably expect that the "situation will reverse in the future," with Waxman lending his weight to them on issues which were not important to him (Davidson and Oleszek 1990, 355).

Waxman was also aided by powerful allies of both parties in the Senate, where his influence on the agenda was minimal. These included: Sen. John Chaffee (R-RI), ranking Republican on the Finance Committee; Sen. Lloyd Bentsen (D-TX), chair of the Finance Committee after 1986; and Sen. John D. Rockefeller IV, chair of the Long Term Care Subcommittee of the Finance Committee. Each of these members favored extending health care benefits to the poor, although their priorities differed somewhat from Waxman's.

The potential sources of resistance to medicaid expansions arose from two groups: those opposed to abortion, who attached crippling amendments to medicaid legislation in 1980, and fiscal conservatives, who dominated the agenda in the early 1980s. Waxman employed both

persuasion and bargaining to establish allies within both camps—
clearing the way for extension in the medicaid program to reach the
agenda.

To pro-lifers, Waxman argued the logic of valuing the life of poor
children through expanding medicaid as an alternative to abortion. He
won over such groups as the Catholic Conference and such
conservative members as Rep. Henry J. Hyde (D-IL) and Sen. Orrin G.
Hatch (R-UT) (Sardell 1991, 28). Hyde called medicaid expansion "a
natural progression." He said, "Once you establish the primacy of life,
you work for those who fall between the cracks." But he also
acknowledged Waxman's skill in gaining his support, adding, "He's
effective as hell" (Morgan 1994a). In addition to persuasion, Waxman
and vital congressional staff worked out a bargain with the Catholic
Conference and Children's Defense Fund to separate the issues of
abortion and medicaid extension (Sardell 1991, 28).

Fiscal conservatives, including many Republicans, such as Sen.
Robert Dole (R-KA) and members of Waxman's own subcommittee,
Rep. William E. Dannemeyer (R-CA) and Thomas J. Tauke (R-IA),
often did not agree with Waxman's agenda. The cost-effective
argument was influential in helping some of these members to safely
support such an expansionary policy. However, given the worsening
health care situation and rising support for government enlargement of
health care financing, fiscal conservatives were not a significant
obstacle at the agenda setting stage. Instead, they exerted their greatest
influence during the adoption phase.

POLICY ADOPTION

Although proposals for medicaid enlargement were considered by
Congress every year except one between 1977 and 1983, this policy
was not adopted until 1984. Beginning in that year and continuing each
year until 1990, Congress passed legislation extending medicaid
eligibility and/or services. Such a dramatic reversal in medicaid 's
treatment could not have been brought about by one individual.
However, Rep. Waxman remained poised and persistent throughout the
entire period, pressing the adoption of medicaid enlargement. Thus, it is
not surprising that when the political and institutional circumstances
changed to favor medicaid's extension, he was successful in gaining
adoption.

Douglas Arnold suggests that once coalition leaders[4] have selected a specific proposal, such as medicaid expansion, they have few potential winning strategies: persuasion, procedural devises, or modification (1990, 88). This section will show how Waxman used all three. However, without the political and institutional changes that occurred during the period, Waxman would not have been as successful. Specifically, without significant changes in medicaid's political support as well as in the budget process and in the norms of federalism, it is unlikely that a policy window would have remained open long enough for Waxman to push through so many expansions.

Procedural Strategies

Waxman recognized the importance of electoral calculations to the success of his proposal. He consistently packaged his extensions of medicaid as part of a larger bill—usually the annual budget reconciliation bill. This strategy was important for several reasons. It helped to decrease the ability of instigators to rouse the attention of the inattentive public and made the role of the individual legislator difficult to trace. Such legislation was virtually veto-proof, safe from filibusters, and protected from most amendments. Therefore, it decreased the number of members he had to win over and increased the chances of congressional support. (See Chapter Six for further discussion of the budget process.)

One of Waxman's most important strategic successes was protecting medicaid from across-the-board cuts mandated by the 1985 Gramm-Rudman-Hollings budget bill. The GRH bill required that all but a few privileged programs be cut in the event that Congress did not deliver a budget that met the deficit target for that year. Although it was one of the final decisions of the budget committee in 1985, the medicaid program was made fully exempt from the cuts. Rep. Buddy MacKay (D-FL), then a member of the Budget Committee, credited Waxman's "persistence, some brinkmanship, and tough bargaining" with winning that agreement (Kosterlitz 1989, 579).

When he was not successful in linking medicaid expansions to the reconciliation bill, he sought other omnibus or high profile measures that could similarly provide cover so members never had to vote directly on the issue of increasing medicaid expenditures. Waxman failed to have the extensions of medicaid included in the fiscal 1988 budget resolution, for example; but through his efforts, they were attached to two other high-priority measures that year—the Family Support Act and the Medicare Catastrophic Coverage Act.

Persuasion

According to Arnold, persuasion involves creating, activating or changing policy preferences of legislators and both the attentive and inattentive publics to fit the original purpose of the coalition leader. The number of individual congressmen that Waxman had to persuade was greatly diminished because of the procedural strategy that he selected— linking medicaid expansions to the "must pass" budget reconciliation bill. This reduced considerably the number of committees involved with the decision and heightened the role that the Democratic party leadership played in the adoption process. The increasingly Democratic composition of the House and Senate during the 1980s made his task easier. The Democratic leadership was largely sympathetic to his goals. By the mid-1980s, the Democratic party had adopted a strategy of "exempting programs for the poor from spending freezes and cuts" (Hook 1985, 1056). The Senate was more of a challenge because fiscal conservatives within both parties exerted more influence than in the House and were more likely to oppose medicaid expansions. Furthermore, his task of persuading the attentive public was also lessened by the changes in the health care policy environment which stimulated bipartisan agreement on the need to address the problems of cost and access.

The nature of the policy and the strategy of attaching extensions to omnibus measures further aided Waxman's ability to persuade, since there were few traceable effects of medicaid expansions which might diminish members' electoral chances. According to Arnold, coalition leaders must consider the electoral effects of their policy on the other members whose support they seek. The increase in medicaid costs was incremental, and nearly half was shifted to a non-voting entity—state governments. Given the changes in the norms of federalism, Congress found it relatively easy to ignore their opposition. Since medicaid's federal financing came from general taxes, its costs were not clearly the result of an identifiable government action.

Many factors facilitated Waxman's task of persuading his colleagues. His generous support of the re-election campaigns of

Democratic members in the House and Senate, especially those of his own committee members, certainly enhanced his persuasive abilities. In addition to his financial resources, his persistence again paid off. Rep. Leon Panetta, former Budget Committee chair, related that "Henry would nag and cajole." He came back repeatedly, asking for more (Morgan 1994a). However, when procedural strategies and persuasion failed, as they often did in conference committee with more conservative Senators, Waxman was prepared with yet another approach—modification.

Modification

In Waxman's arsenal of strategies, modification of his proposal was his last resort. When persuasion failed to win support for his proposal, he modified it, but only when absolutely necessary. In part because of Waxman's persistence, decisions on medicaid often were the last to be decided in conference. Rep. Miller recounted,

> You'd get down to the last negotiations with the conferees, and the last question to be asked would be, "Has Henry signed off?" . . . Those were the most troublesome words to the leadership (Kosterlitz 1989, 580).

And then, if he had to jettison part of his proposal, he would return the next year, seeking to include it. The House-Senate conference on medicaid expansions in 1987 illustrates this pattern. Morgan relates that

> Even the generally more conservative Senate Finance Committee often cooperated with Waxman to expand Medicaid . . . Bentsen a southern centrist Democrat who became chair of the Senate Finance Committee in 1987 repeatedly scaled back or opposed House-backed Medicaid proposals on fiscal grounds. That year he scuttled a House-approved plan to extend Medicaid coverage for a year to those going off welfare, as well as one aimed at preventing the impoverishment of elderly spouses in nursing homes . . . But both provisions were approved the following year . . . (1994a).

Waxman was forced to accept other critical modification in the years 1984 and 1990. He sought to broaden medicaid coverage, but to finance it through a different funding mechanism. Instead of the traditional federal-state shared arrangement, he proposed 100 percent federal financing of the medicaid expansion. The Senate finally agreed to the extensions in eligibility but staunchly opposed changing the funding formula. Waxman relinquished this request and accepted the expansion in benefits. He frequently compromised by scaling down his requests, settling for an incremental change in order to gain passage. But he invariably returned the next year to try again.

CONCLUSION

Waxman played a critical role in facilitating the repeated expansion of medicaid from 1984 to 1990. As the policy entrepreneur, he choreographed the strategy of incrementalism and persistence that exploited the political and institutional circumstances of those years. In this way he maximized enlargements of the medicaid program. His own personal and political resources as chair of the powerful Subcommittee on Health of the HEEC, as possessor of sizable financial resources through his PAC, and as a skillful and tenacious negotiator enabled him to exert extraordinary influence over the policy process in the House and in conference committee. His skill alone can not explain the remarkable series of enlargements in medicaid during the 1980s. Despite his efforts prior to the mid 1980s and after 1990, he was unable to achieve any medicaid enlargements. Had it not been for the important changes in the budget process that reduced the opportunity for amendments, debate and opposition, his success during the mid and late 1980s would have been far more limited. When the budget process was altered again in 1990, new obstacles emerged, once again impeding Waxman's ability to win enactment of medicaid expansions.

Although his role in advancing the cause of medicaid extensions is well-known, Waxman played another important part, in that he helped the states to finance the medicaid mandates they so vehemently opposed. Without his efforts on their behalf, the states would not have found it so easy to obtain generous matching funds from the federal government.

NOTES

1. In 1990, for example, he gave away 43 percent of all money he spent to other Democratic candidates and Democratic party organizations (Morris 1992).

2. In 1977 and 1978, prior to being elected chair to the Subcommittee on Health and the Environment, Waxman supported legislation to expand medicaid.

3. In 1989 and 1990 the states emerged as the only significant opposition to mandatory medicaid expansions.

4. Arnold's definition of coalition leader and Kingdon's policy entrepreneur can be considered interchangeable in this paper. Arnold defines the coalition leader as someone either inside or outside of Congress who: defines problems, shapes alternatives, initiates action, mobilizes support, arranges compromises, and works to see Congress pass specific bills (1990, 88).

PART TWO

The States' Treatment of Medicaid

CHAPTER EIGHT

States' Enlargement of Medicaid: Fiscal Constraints and Divided Government

States complained vociferously about the effect of congressional mandates in boosting medicaid program expenditures during the late 1980s and early 1990s, but they were less forthright in acknowledging their own role in expanding medicaid costs. Changes in state medicaid policies and financing practices contributed importantly to the rapid escalation in costs. After growing at an average rate of 10 percent a year in the early and mid 1980s, state-level medicaid expenditures grew at an average rate of 20.9 percent per year between 1988 and 1992. Researchers have estimated that nearly one-quarter of that growth was attributable to special financing schemes designed by states to maximize medicaid revenues, so that the states' share fell even as their total expenditures rose (Coughlin et al. 1994a, 2, 91).

Severe fiscal strain at the state level, worsened by an accumulation of congressional mandates during the late 1980s, especially those for medicaid, heightened the states' incentives to rely upon cost-shifting strategies to relieve their burden. As a shared program during a time when most federal grants to states were shrinking, medicaid offered states a rare opportunity for increasing the amount of their grants. Although a number of states had engaged in one or another medicaid maximizing strategy since the beginning of the program, the scope and financial impact of state medicaid cost shifting reached unprecedented proportions in the late 1980s and early 1990s. By 1992, thirty-six states had adopted one or more special medicaid financing programs designed to enlarge their federal matching funds (Cromwell et al. 1994, 11-26). Furthermore, a significant portion of medicaid funds derived from these innovative financing mechanisms went into state general funds and were not applied toward medicaid at all (Ku and Coughlin 1995, 46-47).

STATE STRATEGIES FOR SHIFTING COSTS

Shared financing enabled Congress to shift much of the cost of medicaid expansion to the states during the late 1980s and early 1990s. This same feature also enabled the states to leverage billions of dollars from the federal government. Although states have a long history of successfully shaping grants to suit their purposes, open-ended matching grants present particularly tempting opportunities for states to generate additional revenue.[1] In addition, the complexity and flexibility of the medicaid program permit states a great deal of discretion in design of that program (Barrilleaux and Miller 1992; Holahan and Cohen 1986). States exploited these features of medicaid during the late 1980s and early 1990s, using two major strategies: fiscal substitution and special financing mechanisms.

Fiscal Substitution

Fiscal substitution has been a problem common to medicaid and other open-ended matching grants. The lack of a program cap creates especially powerful incentives for states to shift services or clients from one program to another. Such shifting enables them to take advantage of higher matching rates without increasing services. The open-ended nature of medicaid program, its high matching rate (Beam 1980, 141-151)[2], and the scarcity of other open-ended matched programs during the late 1980s and early 1990s made this program especially vulnerable to fiscal substitution.

Shifting a population to medicaid means that the federal government would finance part of the cost of what would otherwise be a fully state-funded service. States have used the medicaid program to finance state health and human service expenses to varying extents since the beginning of the program (Holahan et al. 1993, 33). In the early years of medicaid the number of recipients grew rapidly as states shifted the cost of medical services for the poor from direct state and local spending to medicaid. Incentives to maximize medicaid through shifting costs to the federal government are greatest in those states with broad state-financed human service programs and those with a high federal matching rate (Bovbjerg and Holahan 1982, 18). New York, a state with very broad social welfare coverage, has a long history of aggressively shifting social service programs to medicaid (Stevens and Stevens 1974; Fossett and Wyckoff 1992, 6).

Recently researchers have documented an increase in the use of program shifting, with South Carolina and Missouri among the most active (Gold 1993, 150; Holahan 1992, viii; 1993, 27, 33). A number of statutory changes during the 1980s increased the states' discretion in implementing their medicaid programs, making it easier to shift previously state-funded programs to medicaid (Schneider 1988, 760). Many took advantage of the opportunity. Among the state-federal programs shifted to medicaid during the 1980s were those that had lower matching rates, such as special education, maternal-child health, mental illness, mental retardation and developmental disabilities, substance abuse, home health, and general health assistance (Holahan et al. 1992, viii)

The extension of medicaid services to include home- and community-based care in the early 1980s allowed states to shift personal care services, previously funded through the Title XX Social Services Block Grant Program to medicaid (Holahan 1993, 33). Furthermore, mandated expansions in medicaid eligibility for pregnant women and children were often funded through transferring state maternal child health funding to medicaid agencies. The expansion in EPSDT requirements in 1989 also increased the opportunity for states to shift special education programs operated by school districts to medicaid eligibility (Fossett and Wyckoff 1992, 6). Another costly population that states transferred to medicaid was that of people with AIDS. Whereas care for this group had previously been funded through state general assistance funds, many states sought to make them eligible for SSI (and therefore, medicaid) (Coughlin et al. 1994a, 87).

The extent of this form of cost-shifting is difficult to assess because of a lack of data. Anecdotal accounts abound (General Accounting Office 1991, Surles et al. 1992), but most forms of program shifting can not be accurately estimated because this phenomenon is not measured directly in either of the two major medicaid reporting systems—HCFA 64 and 2082. These forms report medicaid claims and recipients by the type of provider to whom payment is made, not by the service rendered. Consequently, no consensus exists among experts regarding the impact of this form of cost shifting. While the use of program shifting has had an undeniable impact on medicaid's expenditure growth, Coughlin et al. suggest that, "it was probably not very great" (1994a, 88).

Special Financing Programs

Analysts do agree that an important factor in medicaid's growth has been the use of special financing programs, including a combination of provider taxes or donations and disproportionate share payments. These financing schemes vary widely, and states often utilize more than one, but they all seek to increase federal medicaid dollars through non-conventional payment mechanisms. A series of inadvertent and accidental administrative and congressional decisions in the 1980s created a loophole that had the effect of eliminating the state matching requirement. This removed the incentive within states to restrain their medicaid expenditures, and created new possibilities for states to leverage additional funds.

Medicaid was designed as a matching grant, based upon the assumption states would attempt to hold down their expenditures. In congressional testimony in 1991, HCFA administrator Gail Wilensky explained the economic incentives inherent in the shared medicaid program. She testified,

> In a matching program those responsible for expenditure decisions and the direct fiscal management of the program must have a reasonable stake in program costs. The shared responsibility works to shape decisionmaking to contain costs. The requirement for a State share of payment has always acted as a restraint on the otherwise open-ended medicaid program (HECC Subcommittee on Health and the Environment Hearing October 1991, 272).

The loophole that emerged in the late 1980s eliminated this matching requirement and the restraint on state medicaid expenditures. Removing state constraints contributed to rapid growth in medicaid expenditures. Because states were no longer footing their share of the medicaid match, the widespread use of these schemes "resulted in a fundamental restructuring of the medicaid match rate both between federal and state governments as well as across states" according to Holahan et al. (1992, ix). The proportion of medicaid expenditures financed by the federal government is determined by the Federal Medical Assistance Percentage (FMAP).[3] In 1991 the states were able to shift the FMAP from an official average of 57 percent to an actual adjusted average of 61 percent. By 1992, this figure had jumped 12 points to an adjusted 69 percent (Cromwell 1994, 11-35).

The loophole first appeared through a series of inadvertent administrative and congressional decisions. In 1981 Congress created the category of Disproportionate Share Hospitals (DSH), a mechanism for states to pay certain hospitals (those serving a disproportionate number of poor clients) larger than normal medicaid payments. However, most states were slow to implement DSHs because such hospitals generally possessed little political influence in state governments (Morgan 1993c). Some states established such restrictive definitions of DSH in the beginning that few institutions could qualify. Throughout the 1980s Congress repeatedly promoted the use of DSH payments as a means to expand health care financing for the poor. In 1986, it liberalized medicaid payments to institutions serving the poor, allowing states to increase DSH payments even beyond what was permitted by medicare.[4] In 1987 and 1988 Congress set the minimum criteria for defining disproportionate share institutions and established rates at which they must be paid in an attempt to encourage the use of these payments (CBO 1992, 29).

These statutory changes, along with liberal implementation guidelines developed by the Department of Health and Human Services, helped lay a foundation for future financing schemes because they allowed states to target specific hospitals to receive additional medicaid payments. Furthermore, these changes "effectively removed all limitations on payments to disproportionate share hospitals" (CBO 1992, 30). Federal policymakers assumed that the risk of states paying these hospitals extremely generous DSH payments in order to draw a larger medicaid match was quite low because of the necessity for states to come up with their own matching funds.

But a second important action by HCFA removed this restraint on DSH payments. Beginning in 1985, HCFA allowed private funds to be counted as part of the state match for medicaid.[5] It was believed that non-profit agencies, such as United Way, might make modest contributions. However, this decision enabled states to raise their portion of the match from specific health care providers (hospitals, nursing homes, physicians) by taxing or soliciting a donation from them.[6] Variations of this scheme involve the use of intergovernmental transfers or intragovernmental transfers rather than provider payments.[7] By itself, this decision did little to increase the incentive for non-profits or intragovernmental agencies to donate large amounts of money to state medicaid funds. Increasing the pool of funding available for medicaid through taxes and donations would not increase the federal match unless that money was spent on medicaid.

The loophole emerged, however, when states discovered that by combining the use of tax and donation programs with DSH payments they could increase both their medicaid spending and medicaid matching fund at no cost to the state or to the donors. Promising generous DSH payments to specific institutions in return for their donation or tax assured the willing participation of DSH in these financing programs.

West Virginia was the first state to link a voluntary tax program with DSH payments. Hospitals in West Virginia credit Gov. Arch A. Moore, Jr. with originating the idea of using donations from providers to increase medicaid payments to hospitals through DSH payments. That state used its additional medicaid funds to help balance its budget. In 1986 a backlog in unpaid provider claims reached nearly $50 million. West Virginia hospitals voluntarily donated $22.7 million between November 1986 and March 1987 to the state's medicaid program. Consequently, the federal government paid West Virginia $66.4 million for the quarter ending July 30, 1987, helping to balance their medicaid budget (Merrill 1987, 26).

Although DSH payments were of little significance during most of the 1980s, they increased dramatically between 1989 and 1991 when states began linking them with tax and donation programs. From 1989 to 1992, DSH payments exploded, growing from $1 billion to $17 billion (Ku and Coughlin 1995, 30). Although the use of special financing programs among the states varied greatly, the Southeastern states were the first and among the most aggressive. The southeastern DHHS region, which included West Virginia, exceeded all others in the amount of medicaid money generated through taxes, donations and intergovernmental transfers between 1986 and 1992 (Coughlin et al. 1994a, 92). In terms of per capita federal medicaid grants produced by special financing schemes, seven of the top ten states were southern.

These included Alabama, Mississippi, Louisiana, South Carolina, Kentucky, Tennessee, and West Virginia, in the order of per capita funds generated.

Several states took "exceptional advantage" of such financing schemes. New Hampshire stands out as the most egregious of these (Morgan 1993b; Cromwell et al. 1994; Coughlin et al. 1994a). The official federal medicaid matching rate for that state, with its high per capita income, was 50 percent. However, due to its widespread use of financing schemes, the actual matching rate in 1992 rose to an astonishing 159 percent. This figure indicates that New Hampshire succeeded in shifting, not only the total cost of its medicaid program, but a large sum of other state expenditures to the federal government as well. Likewise, Alabama was able to boost its effective federal matching rate from 72 percent to 146 percent in 1992 (Cromwell et al. 1994, 11-31). The total state gain from medicaid financing schemes equaled 25 percent of New Hampshire's general fund in 1993. Louisiana's gain was equivalent to 17 percent; and South Carolina's, 10 percent (Ku and Coughlin 1995, 42).

Little analysis regarding the extent of the DSH program and how the payments were used was available until 1992 when HCFA began requiring reporting of such payments. Studies indicate that the funds were used by health care providers and the states for a variety of purposes. The hospitals often received such generous DSH payments that they were able to finance, not only health care for the poor, but hospital construction and other operational expenses.[8] States also utilized their additional medicaid matching funds in diverse ways, but after reimbursing providers for their donations, most of the "State gains are mixed with other funds and are used broadly throughout the State budgets" (Ku and Coughlin 1995, 39,44).

MOTIVATION FOR STATE FINANCING SCHEMES

The incentive for states to shift costs to the federal government is always present to some extent. But according to James Martin, legislative counsel for the National Governors' Association, the overwhelming reason why states employed medicaid maximizing strategies was "financial necessity" (Interview 1995). During the late 1980s and early 1990s, most states faced severe fiscal strain caused by a number of factors, such as a recession, inadequate state tax structures, a reduction in federal grants-in-aid, and an increase in costly mandates, especially those for medicaid (Gold 1992, 33). Given the constitutional requirement in most states to maintain a balanced budget, and the political limitations on how much taxes could be raised or discretionary spending curtailed, state policymakers eagerly sought alternative sources of revenue. With these pressing financial incentives, many chose to exploit the unique fiscal opportunity the shared medicaid program offered.

Financial incentives were not the only reason states sought to shift medicaid expenditures to the federal government. States were also motivated by a sense of injustice—a violation of the norms of federalism. State officials were frustrated with Congress's apparent disregard for state financial and political circumstances throughout the 1980s. They resented the steady stream of costly mandates imposed by Congress, especially those in medicaid. Kathy Deignan, former Senate Budget Committee aide, reported that after Congress had expanded medicaid for the seventh year in a row, in 1990, "the states were screaming and yelling" (Interview 1995). Having been rebuffed in their attempt to persuade Congress to stop further medicaid mandates, the states sought to satisfy their grievance through other means—shifting the cost of medicaid mandates back to the federal government.

Financial Incentives

Analysts have long recognized the incentive within states to maximize the benefit of a grant by shaping its use to conform to their own priorities (Tiebout 1956). Because of competitive pressures, states seek to provide an attractive array of services at least cost to their citizens. The strength of this incentive, however, varies among states and over time. These incentives to pursue cost-shifting strategies arise from various sources, including the extent of fiscal strain in the state and the strength of political opposition to raising taxes or cutting programs to balance the budget.

The incentive to exploit federal grants rises with financial stress. Peterson and Wong analyze this phenomenon. They write,

> The more resources are strained, the greater the politicians' desire to use federal dollars to solve local problems and the less their willingness to use local funds to help smooth over administrative

difficulties. Prosperous, growing communities see federal aid as a supplement to their own resources that can help them achieve goals they could not undertake on their own. Deteriorating communities see federal aid as a means for ameliorating their problems, and they resist those regulations that limit local flexibility (1986, 19).

In studying state responses to fiscal strain in the early 1980s, Durman likewise found that financial stress exerts a significant impact upon states' willingness to engage in the grant maximizing behavior of shifting non-subsidized programs to subsidized ones. [9] He observes:

A state will shift its pattern of response as it moves from a situation of moderate strain to one of extreme stress . . . [U]nder mild strain governments engage in a wide variety of incremental measures designed to relieve the immediate crisis without radically altering the allocation among programs. Reducing surpluses, tax increases, accounting changes, optimistic budgeting, hiring freezes, etc., are characteristic responses in the early stages of a fiscal crisis . . . As the crisis deepens or is prolonged, the state must shift its attention to major programmatic shifts . . . [T]here is a point at which immediate fiscal issues dominate all other concerns (1981, 27).

The objective measures of a state's fiscal capacity may not reflect the level of fiscal strain in a particular state, however, because particularly strong political opposition to tax increases may limit the options of state policymakers. The influence of political factors in defining "fiscal strain" within a state therefore contributes to great variation among the states in their willingness to shift costs to the federal government (Durman, 1981, 36).

Beginning in the late 1980s, many states "began a period of sharp fiscal decline" (Miller 1993, 119) that played a major role in shaping state incentives to find politically acceptable means of increasing their revenue. In 1990, 33 states faced budget deficits (Hinds 1990, E5). The National Association of State Budget Officers reported at the end of 1991 that 22 states had balances of less than one percent of spending in general funds and rainy day funds as a proportion of annual general-fund spending. Average balances among the states equaled 1.5 percent—the lowest since the recession of 1983 (Gold 1992, 34).

An increase in expenditures over which the states had little control contributed greatly to their fiscal stress. Of 11 factors identified by Steven D. Gold as sources of state stress in 1991, the federal government played a role in seven (1992, 33). Health care expenditures were one of the most significant, and medicaid was the item which increased most rapidly. Their burden grew from 9 percent of the states' general fund in 1989 to 12 percent in 1992. Gold contends that, "The growth of Medicaid spending is not the only source of state fiscal stress, but it is perhaps the largest single cause [of prospective deficits in the states]" (1993, 133-135).

A number of factors were instrumental in raising the cost of medicaid. In addition to the series of congressional mandates from 1984 to 1990, other factors outside of the states' control included growth in the number of the uninsured, the increasing incidence of AIDS, medical inflation, and lawsuits and the threat of lawsuits related to the Boren Amendments.

The Boren amendments guaranteed that hospitals and nursing homes would be reimbursed at rates that are "reasonable and adequate to meet the costs which must be incurred by efficiently and economically operated facilities" (OBRA 1980 and 1981). These statutes invited health care providers to sue states for higher reimbursement rates, which have meant "states are under increasing legal pressure to raise [medicaid] payment rates" (Holahan et al. 1993, 32).[10] The increase in medicaid reimbursement as well as the cost of litigation associated with the Boren Amendments has been considerable. Because of Boren-related suits, Pennsylvania estimates its medicaid expenditures increased by 15 percent; Washington state hospital reimbursement rates grew by 9 percent; and Virginia was ordered to reimburse hospitals a total of $120 million over four years (Anderson and Scanlon 1993, 88-89).

What made this growth in medicaid expenditures so serious was that the states' ability to raise revenue did not keep up. Although revenue growth lagged behind medicaid costs throughout the 1980s, the situation grew worse after 1988. Medicaid expenditures increased at 18.7 percent per year between 1988 and 1991, while state revenues crept ahead at only 6.5 percent annually (Coughlin et al. 1994a, 82).[11] Consequently, the increase in medicaid expenditures above the states' ability to raise revenues placed intense strain on state budgets.

Several other factors also stretched state budgets during the 1980s. The legacy of OBRA 1981 meant federal aid to the states declined from $127.6 billion in 1980 to $119.7 billion in 1990 in constant dollars (ACIR 1992, 60). As federal aid decreased, it also became more concentrated. Medicaid became the dominant source of state grant revenue, increasing from 17.2 percent of all federal grants-in-aid in 1980 to approximately 42 percent in 1992 (ACIR 1992, 61). While federal grants were shrinking during the 1980s, so was the states' ability to generate revenue from traditional tax sources. Neither sales nor corporate taxes performed very well during this period, according to Gold (1993, 139). He attributes this phenomenon to changes in the structure of the U.S. economy, which has become increasingly service-oriented, and the persistence of relatively slow economic growth. Although states had had trouble generating revenue during the 1980s, the recession of 1990 abruptly worsened the situation. The performance of three of the most important sources of state income—general, personal, and corporate taxes—declined even further in 1990 and 1991 (Gold 1993, 140-141).

Most states do not undertake grant maximizing strategies, such as program shifting, until other approaches to relieve fiscal strain have been implemented, or unless the period of stress is prolonged (Durman 1981, 30). By the early 1990s most states had sustained economic strain for several years. This meant that a number of short term strategies for decreasing costs and increasing revenues had already been exhausted. Between 1985 and 1990 most states had enacted a "modest" net increase in income taxes (Gold 1993, 142). As fiscal pressures mounted, thirty states enacted further tax increases totaling $10.3 billion in 1990, and $15 billion in 1991 (Claiborne 1992; Pierce 1991, 1008).

State officials took steps to slow spending for many services during the late 1980s, but nevertheless found it necessary to cut back even further during the early 1990s. Gold reports that, "all categories of the budget were adversely affected" (1993, 138). 29 states cut more than $8 billion from their 1991 budgets (Pierce 1991, 1008). Higher education was one of the hardest hit (Gold 1993, 138). Schools and welfare benefits also suffered (Fossett and Wyckoff 1992). And, although corrections continued to expand, its rate of growth decreased. In addition, state employees went without raises in 23 states in 1992 (Gold, 1993, 139).

Although necessary to balance state budgets, these strategies were not politically popular. Jane Horvath, director of the American Public Welfare Association, stated,

> The point is that states have raised taxes, and they've raised a bunch this year and last. There's a limit to what you can do. The White House is well aware of the limits of having to raise taxes. And I think the public holds local officials far more accountable for this stuff (quoted in Haas 1991, 1806).

Her point was illustrated in New Jersey. That state raised taxes in 1990, which sparked a "popular revolt that rocked the states polling booths last November and spooked politicians everywhere," according to one report from 1991 (Mandel et al. 1991, 26). State officials felt tremendous pressure to find new and creative ways of raising additional revenue without such political costs. Maximizing the amount of federal revenue through manipulating the medicaid program emerged as the only option available to the states during the early 1990s (Coughlin et al. 1994b, 861).

Those states with the greatest financial strain were the first and among the most energetic in establishing these financing programs. West Virginia, the first state to institute a special financing plan, was especially strapped financially in 1986. Other southern states also suffered serious fiscal strain, in part because of the burden of the congressional mandates to expand medicaid coverage. Victor Miller explains that these states often had "smaller Medicaid benefit packages, less intrusive state oversight of providers, less expansive AFDC and SSI eligibility, and a higher share of families with incomes under the poverty line" than the national average (1993, 124). Therefore, the mandates imposed larger costs upon these states, requiring sizable increases in their programs. Between 1986 and 1992 all southern states, except South Carolina, implemented extensions in medicaid coverage that exceeded the national average (Cromwell et al. 1994, 11-32). One survey conducted in 1992 found that in the 13 southern states, medicaid mandates cost $1.9 billion in 1991 and $1.5 billion in 1992 (Wnuk 1993, 13).

Not only did Southern states suffer disproportionately from the medicaid mandates, they also had the most to gain from exploiting the federal match. Their low per capita income levels meant these states possessed the highest average matching rate of any region in the country. Excluding Virginia, which did not implement a special financing program, the average FMAP among 11 Southern states equaled 70.7 in 1990, whereas the national average was 59.9 (*Medicaid Source Book* 1993, 485-486).[12]

Outside the Southeastern region, states whose fiscal circumstances were not objectively as strained also aggressively pursued medicaid financing schemes. New Hampshire exceeded all others in this regard. Cromwell et al. suggest that financial strain played an important role in New Hampshire's pursuit of medicaid as a source of state revenue. They point out that between 1988 and 1991 New Hampshire expanded its tax effort more than any other state (Cromwell et al. 1994, 11-34). However, they fail to note that New Hampshire ranked fifth among the states in its tax capacity in 1988; and despite this financial advantage, it exerted the lowest level of tax effort (with no sales or income tax) among all the states from 1980 to 1990 (Gold 1993, 146-147). Furthermore, unlike the southern states, it was not substantially affected by the medicaid mandates (Cromwell et al. 1994, 11-34). New Hampshire obviously possessed greater potential to raise revenue than its politicians were willing to tap. This suggests the fiscal strain felt by New Hampshire policymakers was related to their political priorities.

Morgan explains the political circumstances that influenced New Hampshire policymakers. He writes,

> With the New Hampshire primary only months away and [Gov. Judd Gregg (R)] planning to run for the U.S. Senate as a fiscal conservative, the possibility of imposing an income tax or sales tax was not seriously considered ... Since 1972, no candidate for governor has been elected without first taking a pledge to oppose any new broad-based tax ...
>
> On Nov.12, the legislature, meeting in one-day special session, easily approved the change. The House margin was 283-42 and the Senate approved it 19-3.
>
> One House member voting against it was Rep. William Riley (D) ... "I thought it was despicable," he said. "We don't need to dip into this Medicaid scam because we haven't tapped one of the biggest sources there is: the income tax" (1993b).

Massachusetts was also among the top ten users of special financing programs. Like New Hampshire, it had a large relative increase in tax effort between 1988 and 1992, reflecting some fiscal strain. However, unlike New Hampshire, Massachusetts possessed one of the highest per capita medicaid expenditures in the nation and already had one of the highest levels of tax effort (Cromwell et al. 1994, 11-28—11-32; Gold 1993, 147).[13] Clearly, great differences existed in the priorities of both states; yet, each chose to institute a medicaid financing scheme because of potentially large benefits to be gained and the lack of political costs associated with that policy.

Although 36 states had implemented special financing programs by the end of 1992, fourteen other states,[14] some of which expanded tax effort well beyond the national average (e.g., Connecticut and New Jersey), had not. And of those that did institute a financing scheme, the amount of federal money they leveraged varied greatly (Cromwell et al. 1994, 11-32). Although this evidence is strong that financial strain has encouraged special financing strategies, other political variables, including political culture, no doubt played a role. Derthick cites the importance of this factor in shaping incentives within states to shift program costs. She writes,

> In states that tend to be receptive to government action in general and that have no ideological bias against federal action in particular, the charge of "not taking advantage of federal funds" or of "failing to meet federal standards" is potentially very damaging to politicians. In other states, where government activity in general and federal activity in particular are more resisted, the risks of nonparticipation or defiance are lower (1970, 215).

While the influence of political culture may help to explain why several states did not respond to the financial incentives inherent in the medicaid financing strategies, this is an area that bears further research.

Abuse of Federalism

Besides financial incentives, another factor was influential in promoting the extensive use of medicaid financing schemes—the widespread frustration among state officials with Congress and its increasing use of mandates. In 1989, as the states faced rising fiscal strain, they pleaded with Congress in a public display of unity to stop imposing costly medicaid mandates upon them. James Martin of the NGA remarked that in twenty years, he had never seen the states "more unified on any issue" (Interview 1995). Nevertheless, their appeals were ignored as Congress adopted further mandatory expansions in each of its next two reconciliation bills. Such blatant disregard for the state governments prompted states to seek alternate routes to protect themselves from the fiscal effects of congressional actions.

State officials displayed their outrage during this period, using such terms as, "fieldhands of federalism," "shift and shaft federalism," and "fend-for-yourself federalism" (Farney and Davidson 1989; Peirce 1991, 1008; Gold 1993, 36). Shortly after Congress rejected the appeal of the NGA in September 1989, Governor James Blanchard (D-MI) complained that, "Washington has gone from revenue sharing to revenue bleeding" (quoted in Farney and Davidson 1989).

A number of states began launching political strategies to get Washington lawmakers to be more accountable to them. Many state officials met individually or in regional groups with their congressional delegations to protest the fiscal impact of mandates. Five state legislatures passed resolutions urging Congress to stop passing costs to the states.

Some states have taken even bolder steps. Reports have surfaced that some state legislators were relying upon the redrawing of congressional districts after the 1990 census to gain policy concessions from their congressional delegations (Krane 1993, 147). Reminiscent of the era before the 17th Amendment when state legislatures elected their U.S. senators, Alabama's state legislators unanimously adopted a resolution in 1992 requesting members of their congressional delegation to "appear before a joint session of the Legislature to discuss the problems of unfunded federal mandates" (Wnuk 1993, 13). South Dakota adopted a similar measure; and 14 other states were considering doing the same. Although states cannot demand that their congressional delegation appear, ignoring such a request would carry significant political costs (Claiborne 1993).

One analyst suggested that states believed the questionable medicaid financing techniques were *poetic justice* for what Congress had imposed upon them (Haas 1991, 1804). Although the financial incentives inherent in the medicaid financing programs were a prominent factor in promoting their widespread adoption, growing resentment toward Congress may also have been a consideration. Through shifting the financial burden of special medicaid financing programs, states were also shifting responsibility for imposing intrusive mandates back to the federal government. Correcting what they perceived to be an injustice may well have served as a powerful motivator among many state-level officials.

FACTORS AFFECTING THE STATES' IMPLEMENTATION OF FINANCING SCHEMES

The opportunity for states to exploit the shared medicaid program through innovative cost-shifting strategies existed because of a loophole in the medicaid law; and states moved quickly to exploit that opportunity. What remains to be explained is, how did so many states manage to design and implement such diverse and complex changes in their medicaid financing programs so rapidly? And, in light of the billions of dollars the states were able to leverage from the federal government over several years, why did federal officials not act more promptly to stop them?

Political and bureaucratic factors are critical in explaining state responses to federal grants. Improved administrative and political capacity at the state level helped to facilitate the widespread adoption of financing schemes. Another important factor that determines the way states use federal grants is the nature of conflict between and within the various levels of government (Bardach 1977; Pressman and Wildavsky 1973). Conflict between branches at the national level and an important, but little recognized, alliance between states and Congress was critical in promoting the practice of innovative financing schemes. To understand how the states leveraged billions of federal dollars through the medicaid program during the early 1990s, it is therefore necessary to examine the administrative and political developments within each level of government and between levels of government.

State-level political and administrative factors

A number of factors helped to facilitate the widespread adoption of these financing programs. These include the nature of political alliances that emerged in support of the policy, the character of the political process determining medicaid financing, and changes in the political and administrative expertise of policymakers and public interest groups.

Assuming that state politicians seek to maximize their utility while minimizing their costs (Grogan 1993, 3), special medicaid financing programs offered them the ideal policy. These schemes brought additional revenue into the state, especially targeted to a narrow interest group, health care providers, at no apparent cost to the taxpayers of the state. Verdier summarizes the winners and losers of this policy as follows:

> The winners in this situation were the providers—who got back the amount they paid in taxes and, often, increased Medicaid reimbursement as well—and states—who were able to pay for increased Medicaid and other states expenditures without paying any of the political costs of raising taxes or cutting spending in other areas of the budget. The loser was, of course, the federal government, which ended up paying out more and more in federal Medicaid matching funds (1993, 523).

By concentrating benefits on an important, well-organized constituency, and by shifting the cost of doing so to the federal government, state policymakers promoted a strong alliance in support of these financing schemes, while creating no opposition.

The character of medicaid policymaking was another important factor that promoted the use of such strategies. Although the policymaking process differs among the states with regard to the level of discretion awarded the administration and the dispersion of authority among different departments, important program designs are monitored by only a small contingent of the public (Barilleaux and Miller 1992, 99). Health care providers tend to be vigilant over medicaid matters that affect them, such as benefit policy; and constituents (especially the elderly) are concerned with eligibility and coverage (Grogan 1993). Matters related to reimbursing health care providers and securing a greater federal match would be expected to hold little interest for most of the general public. Therefore, the majority within a state were unlikely to be aware of the change in medicaid policy that instituted the special financing program. The lack of public knowledge, interest, and understanding of the complexity of medicaid financing contributed to the absence of public scrutiny, which narrowed the sphere of actors involved in the decision to adopt this policy.

Although the broad distribution of benefits and the absence of financial costs to the state meant significant opposition to adopting special medicaid financing programs was not likely, the lack of public scrutiny certainly assisted in the speedy adoption of these policies. Had the public been more fully informed, some might have objected to these schemes on grounds of fairness or the appearance of engaging in questionable practices. In fact, in New Hampshire 42 members of the House and 3 members of the state Senate opposed the medicaid cost-shifting plan supported by the Republican leadership (Morgan 1993b). State Representative Bill Seliff, (R-NH) opposed the measure, despite his loyalty to his home state and to his party. He stated,

> My basic concern was that the federal government was getting screwed. We balanced the [state] budget with this loophole. I don't think the federal government can continue to run this way (quoted in Morgan 1993b).

Had this issue received greater public scrutiny, more opposition may have emerged within a number of states.

Another factor that promoted the use of special financing schemes was the enhanced political and administrative potential of state-level governments. In order to take advantage of the medicaid financing schemes, states had to design and coordinate at least two programs: a DSH program and a tax and/or donation program while appeasing the affected providers and meeting HCFA regulations for the program. Many states implemented more than one type of program in order to maximize their revenue. Without skilled administrators and politicians, states would not have been able to design, coordinate, and implement these programs.

Since the 1960s the role of patronage has diminished within state governments, helping to usher in a transformation of personnel. The level of expertise and sophistication among state workers has risen (Derthick 1987, 72; Nathan 1993, 16; Rivlin 1992, 104). More sophisticated staff has been an important factor in promoting the exploitation of federal grants, including complex schemes such as that for medicaid.

Examining state responses to cutbacks in federal assistance during the early 1980s, Durman found that the "relative size and sophistication of the administrative apparatus . . . are indicative of a state's ability to implement complex intertitle transfers, or to actively shape its policy direction . . . "(1981, 40). Whereas exploiting the fungibility of medicaid through intertitle transfers is an old game for most of the states, devising creative financing strategies that would meet HCFA approval and appease the various state level constituencies required a high level of quantitative and analytical skills.

In addition to developments within state governments, the intergovernmental lobby also increased its capacity over the past several decades (Beer 1977; Derthick 1987, 69; Hall 1989, 31). This development enhanced the use of special medicaid financing in two important ways: it promoted rapid diffusion of the financing strategies among the states and it helped them defend the strategy at the national level.

Beer defines the lobby as consisting of "governors, mayors, county supervisors, city managers, and other officeholders, usually elective, who exercise general responsibilities in state and local government" (1977, 11). Not only have these officeholders become more active in policymaking at the national level as individual representatives of their governments, but the non-governmental institutions of federalism or public interest groups[15] have grown in influence as well. Krane writes,

> The increasingly competitive interdependence of national and state governments has spawned a significant growth in Washington-based associations that represent the interests of the states. Governors, other state elected officials, and state administrators transcend their institutional authority and extend their influence over national policymaking through membership in these so-called public interest groups . . . State administrators, like all public administrators, find themselves choosing or being forced to play politics (1993, 152-153).

Although five of the largest public interest groups are best-known for their lobbying, they spend more than half of their budgets on nonlobbying activities.[16] These organizations focus their energies and resources on "research, publication, training, and service efforts for their members and clients" (Wright 1988, 282-283). Such activities have helped promote the spread of innovative financing programs through creating formal and informal lines of communication among state-level officials organizations. Jim Martin, legislative counsel for the NGA, emphasized the importance of sharing information among colleagues. He noted, "Governors openly admit they steal ideas from each other. It is one of the things they do best" (Interview 1995). State medicaid directors also "exchange ideas over the telephone about how to finance their programs" (Haas 1991, 1807).

Sharing of information regarding how to maximize medicaid funds through cost-shifting strategies helped states that had not had previous experience with such strategies. Morgan describes how other states assisted New Hampshire.

> That March [1991], [state Rep. Donna P. Sytek, former chairman of the New Hampshire House Ways and Means Committee] said, she heard about a loophole in Medicaid law at a conference of state legislators. "They've got this little scheme and you can use it [the federal money] for highways," she quoted a Missouri legislator as telling her . . . others in state government were thinking along the same lines. [Republican state senator Douglas E. Hall] recalled that someone had brought him an article about Massachusetts's use of the loophole, and Sytek said an official in state Health and Social Services Commissioner Harry Bird's office also "had discovered the loophole, bless his heart"(1993b).

Intergovernmental lobbying organizations promoted the use of special financing programs through advocating the state position at the national level of government. Unsuccessful in winning HCFA's approval of special financing programs, the states appealed to others in the legislative and executive branches. Although their lobby was not consistently successful in its attempts to win congressional support—it conspicuously failed to persuade Congress stop medicaid mandates—it achieved remarkable success in winning congressional support in its battle with HCFA over medicaid financing regulations.

Numerous state officials and representatives of public interest groups appealed to members of Congress to defend the use of special financing programs throughout the late 1980s and early 1990s. At HECC and SFC hearings regarding the state-financing of medicaid in September, October, and November 1991, for example, the National

Governors' Association, National Conference of State Legislatures, and the National Association of Counties testified.

These state officials lobbied the White House as well as Congress. In 1991 a series of private negotiations took place between the Bush administration and the NGA on the matter of state financing of medicaid (Morgan 1994b). The approach of the 1992 presidential election gave important governors added leverage. Bush felt pressure to maintain friendly relations with them. Morgan related how Governor Schaefer of Maryland won concessions from the White House just prior to that race. He writes,

> On Oct. 9, 1992, however, after Gov. William Donald Schaefer appealed personally to Bush, in telephone calls and writing, HHS freed $75 million in disputed federal Medicaid payments for Maryland. Schaefer, a Democrat, endorsed Bush four days before the Nov. 3 election (1994b).

He also describes another such incident.

> On Nov. 14, 1991, OMB Associate Director Scully held a teleconference with six Republican governors who pleaded for relief from the OMB proposal [for new regulations limiting the use of state financing schemes]. "They were saying they'd have to call their legislatures back and it would be a political catastrophe for them," Scully recalled in an interview before leaving government (1994b).

Federal Institutional and Political Factors

The states' ability to exploit medicaid through innovative financing schemes was facilitated by a number of institutional and political factors at the national level as well. The arrangement of shared powers among the branches of government, which enabled one branch to subvert the policy goals of another, was critical. During the late 1980s and early 1990s the difference in goals between the executive and legislative branches of government regarding the medicaid program was aggravated by divided government. The political incentives of members of Congress to perform constituency service, regardless of party affiliation, also played a central role in promoting the states' use of these schemes.

After examining rulemaking and policymaking for the medicaid program during the 1980s, Kinney concluded that the situation in which institutions that must share powers are controlled by different parties constitutes a "deep structural problem" for our government (Kinney 1990, 901; Stone 1991, 12). Kinney describes the difference in goals between the executive and legislative branches that existed during the 1980s as follows:

> The problems with Medicaid rule and policymaking since 1981 stem in large part from a political tug of war between Congress and the Executive Branch about the scope and mission of the Medicaid program in terms of eligible groups as well as benefit and payment levels. The Executive Branch has been chiefly concerned with limiting federal financial commitment to the Medicaid program . . . Congress clearly has a more expansive vision of the Medicaid program and is more inclined to exert federal control over policy on eligibility, benefits and their coverage and payment to providers (1990, 900).

During the late 1980s and early 1990s, this *tug of war* between the branches and between parties continued as members of the Democratic Congress repeatedly thwarted the efforts of the Republican-controlled administration to limit medicaid financing schemes.

Chubb points out two ways in which Congress exerts influence over the administration of federal grants: through the power the oversight committees extend over the administrative agencies and through the "selective influence of members" on behalf of their constituents (1985, 1009). These methods of influence help explain how Congress was instrumental in promoting the state use of medicaid financing mechanisms. First, dominated by a Democratic majority, the oversight committees helped to engineer legislation that blocked HCFA from issuing new regulations to limit the states' special financing schemes. And second, after this strategy was no longer feasible, members of Congress sought to gain concessions and exceptions for their home states.

When West Virginia designed its innovative DSH and voluntary donation program in 1986, HCFA initially approved the plan, but then reversed its decision. Thereafter, it struggled against the judicial and then the legislative branches to limit the use of such programs. A DHHS appeals board at first upheld HCFA's disallowance of West Virginia's donation program in 1986; and HCFA announced its intention to modify the regulations to further limit taxes and donations from health care providers (Haas 1991, 1806; CBO 1992, 32). A federal district court overturned this decision, however, which in turn was upheld on appeal. State financing schemes were declared legal. Because of the fear of widespread use of these strategies and the potential fiscal impact, HCFA continued to attempt to devise regulations limiting their use. Some Democrats in Congress suggest political motives prompted HFCA as well.

One of Waxman's staff suggests that the administration's lack of support for DSH in general, and HCFA's foot-dragging in the implementation of that program throughout the early 1980s, fueled "distrust" between the branches. He claims that proponents of medicaid expansions in Congress feared a fiscally-minded HCFA might gut the DSH program if given the opportunity. This ideological tension between the executive and legislative branches prompted Congress to protect DSH. From 1988 through 1990, Congress adopted annual moratoria prohibiting HCFA from issuing regulations pertaining to the states' financing mechanisms. While a lack of trust was part of the explanation for the moratoria, another more pragmatic reason might have motivated Congress. The Democratically-controlled Congress wished to facilitate the cash-strapped states' ability to implement the costly medicaid expansions it had already enacted and planned to continue enacting. It ignored state pleas to desist from mandates, while protecting the states' opportunity to pay for them with federal money. These were mandates with money—through a back door.

This matter did not attract much attention because it initially was limited to only a few states.[17] It generated little debate in Congress. Using omnibus legislation for protection, Henry Waxman repeatedly won approval of the moratorium in the House Energy and Commerce Committee, and ushered it through Congress relatively hidden. Morgan writes,

> . . . the efforts [of the Bush administration to issue regulations] were blocked by Rep. Waxman, who was unconvinced that abuses were widespread and wanted to help hospitals overwhelmed by uninsured

patients, such as public hospitals serving thousands of immigrants in his home Los Angeles County (1994b).

Over time, this issue gained increased visibility and significance. In 1990 budget negotiations, Waxman blocked "key elements" of the Bush administration's plan to curtail state schemes. However, he "acquiesced to phasing out the use of 'donations' to fund payments to hospitals." This created an urgency for states who had not already done so, to jump on the medicaid "gravy train" (Morgan 1994b).

During 1991, this issue took on additional urgency for both the administration and Congress for several reasons. The size and scope of the financing schemes mushroomed in that year, when 28 additional states (making a total of 34) began implementing these programs. The costs of medicaid also escalated from an 18.8 percent annual growth rate in 1989 to 26.7 percent in 1990 (Coughlin et al. 1994a, 93). Congress was surprised in 1991, because they were kept in the dark without adequate data regarding the scope of the states' use of these programs, according to one Waxman aide.

This aide further claims that perhaps one reason for the delay in providing information to Congress was because the White House was partly responsible for the growth in medicaid expenditures. He asserts that officials in the White House helped to facilitate the use of financing schemes in specific states, such as New Hampshire, in order to enhance Republican political objectives.[18] However, the magnitude of the states use of these financing schemes also caught OMB off guard. Morgan reports,

> It was late March of 1991, when top aides trooped into a meeting with Budget Director Richard G. Darman in a spacious suite in the Old Executive Office Building with some bad news. They informed him that quarterly reports just coming in from the 50 states indicated that the budget he had sent to Congress two months earlier had underestimated federal spending on Medicaid by billions of dollars.
>
> A "ballistic" Darman "wanted to know how this could possibly happen," recalled a former aide. "How could we not know about this? He was outraged . . . how could our numbers be so bad? . . . "
>
> In July, a "SWAT team" made up of budget experts from Darman's Office of Management and Budget (OMB) and the Department of Health and Human Services concluded that a principal

reason for the unexpected [medicaid] cost run-up was the fact that states were using "schemes" and "devices" to increase federal Medicaid grants, primarily through the disproportionate share hospitals program (1994b).

If key administration officials had known of the widespread use of these strategies sooner, they might have taken a more active role in limiting them. The financial impact of these measures earned them a higher priority among the administration in late 1991. Thomas Scully, a top OMB health policy official, met with the governors during the summer of that year to explain the administration's new tougher stance on medicaid financing programs. According to Haas,

> Scully's high-profile involvement underscores the Administration's concern about the states' medicaid financing innovations. If it was merely a dispute over medical rules, HCFA would probably handle the matter alone. But the skyrocketing of medicaid costs prompted OMB director Darman and HHS secretary Louis W. Sullivan in late April to announce a "management review" of the program (1991, 1807).

The issue became more visible and contentious in Congress as well because of the Budget Enforcement Act of 1990. According to that legislation, if Congress successfully blocked HCFA's regulations in 1991 and medicaid expenditures continued their rapid escalation, Congress would be forced to cut $5 billion from other entitlements or confront a sequester (Kimball 1991; Rich 1991).[19] This dilemma for congressional advocates brought an end to congressional moratoria on HCFA medicaid regulations. The oversight committees held a number of hearings on the issue in 1991. Despite testimony from many states, health care representatives, and advocates for the poor, and the strong support of many members of the House and Senate oversight committees, Congress ultimately was unable to pass legislation that would block HCFA from issuing regulations. Such regulations took effect on January 1, 1992.

The failure of Congress to achieve consensus on this issue did not stop individual members from protecting important interests, such as hospitals, and their home states. Many legislators sought last minute amendments to medicaid legislation or through negotiations with

HCFA to allow exceptions for their home states. Such interventions were not limited to the liberal members of Congress, nor to members of the oversight committees. Affected interest groups are especially cognizant of new awards of federal money, which influences them to evaluate members of Congress more favorably (Stein and Bickers 1994, 394). The fact that powerful health care interest groups benefited from such schemes no doubt encouraged many members to act, regardless of their fiscal tendencies. Morgan illustrates the strength of the incentive to assist the home district through several examples:

> Arkansas' tax on health care providers was permitted to remain in effect until June 1993, as a result of quick action by Sen. David H. Pryor (D-Ark). A date change protected West Virginia, New Hampshire, and Wisconsin . . . Alabama and other states were given until October 1992 to revise they way they financed their Medicaid programs (1994b).

Morgan further elaborates on New Hampshire's example:

> New Hampshire Sen. Warren Rudman (R) inserted provisions in a key Medicaid bill during the final hours of the congressional session at the end of 1991 to protect New Hampshire's Medicaid scheme through June of 1993. A co-author of the Gramm-Rudman-Hollings deficit reduction law, Rudman said recently that he had no regrets about his role. My attitude was that if that's the way the game is played, we'll play it too," he said. "If we were going to have this loophole, I wasn't going to see New Hampshire stand idly by" (1993b).

In addition to taking legislative action, legislators negotiated with the administration to obtain favors. Morgan writes,

> Senate Majority Leader George J. Mitchell (D-Maine), making it clear to his colleagues that he was on the floor speaking for his state, recorded an administration letter promising that Maine's program could continue through June 1992 . . . In March 1992, Arizona's Republican Gov. J. Fife Symington III, accompanied by both Arizona senators and Rep. Jim Kolbe (R-Ariz), met with top OMB and HHS officials at the Roosevelt Room in the White House to ask for relief

from the impact of the 1991 statute. Three months later the administration gave Symington about half of what he wanted (1994b).

The sharing of powers between branches at the national level meant that Congress could thwart the administration. This case illustrates the influence that Congress exerts on medicaid policymaking. Chubb captures the significance of political factors in the administration of federal grants, saying, "weak enforcement and local domination, which may be interpreted as failure, may also be what Washington wants for a particular program in a particular place and time" (1985, 1011). This is precisely what Congress wanted during the late 1980s and early 1990s. Despite the opposition of the executive branch, and under pressure from powerful health care interest groups and the states, Congress intervened to promote the states' ability to raid the federal treasury.

CONCLUSION

Despite their claims to be victims of cost-shifting, the states proved that they could also be effective perpetrators. Under intensifying financial pressures, caused in part by a stream of federal mandates during the 1980s, and aided by a loophole in the medicaid law, the states shift billions of dollars from the federal treasury to their own. For several years, a Democratic Congress succeeded in blocking the Republican administration's attempts to limit the states' use of this strategy. Furthermore, once regulations became inevitable, individual members of both parties in Congress sought to please important constituents and their home states through last minute action that extended the use of these programs. Because of the states' widespread use of these innovative financing schemes, total medicaid expenditures mushroomed in the early 1990s.

NOTES

1. Martha Derthick analyzed one of the most egregious examples of this phenomenon in which states exploited the vague language of social services grants in the early 1970s, enabling them to generate billions of additional dollars from the federal government (1975).

2. The medicaid Federal Medical Assistance Percentages (FMAP) or matching rate, ranges from 50 to 83 percent. This is very generous compared to many other grants. In fiscal year 1992, ten states had FMAPs between 50 and 60 percent; 15 states had rates between 60 and 70 percent; and 14 states had rates greater than 70 percent (*Medicaid Source Book* 1993, 484).

3. FMAP = 100 percent minus the state share; the state share = state per capita income^2/per capita income^2 x .45.

4. Prior to OBRA 1986, aggregate medicaid payments to hospitals could not exceed what medicare would have paid.

5. Prior to that time, private funds had been limited to the state share of training funds.

6. Depending on the state federal matching rate, each dollar of donated or taxed money could generate between one and four dollars of federal matching funds.

7. *Intergovernmental transfers* include transfers from local governments to the state for medicaid. They often come from areas with locally funded public hospitals with heavy medicaid and charity patient loads. *Intragovernmental transfers* are those that one state agency gives to another to be used for medicaid. These funds are used to increase the match and are then spent for care delivered at state-owned hospitals, such as state psychiatric hospitals or state university teaching hospitals.

8. Hospitals reported using these funds for a variety of activities, including: providing services to AIDS patients and capital expenditures, such as developing a new clinic, purchasing an ambulance or replacing old radiology equipment. At one hospital the funds enabled it to obtain a commercial loan from a bank. Others placed the funds in interest-bearing trusts (Ku and Coughlin 1995, 39).

9. Durman examined state responses to federal cutbacks in medicaid and other social services programs in 1981. Although he explores the phenomenon of "intertitle transfer" and fungibility, I hold that the factors influencing states to pursue these medicaid maximizing strategies are not significantly different from those promoting states to develop medicaid financing schemes later in the decade.

10. Hospitals or nursing homes in California, Connecticut, Michigan, Missouri, New York, Pennsylvania, Texas, Virginia, and Washington successfully brought suit against the state to increase medicaid reimbursement rates to conform to the requirements of the Boren Amendments. In a number of other states, fear of litigation has prompted states to increase reimbursement rates (Anderson and Scanlon 1993, 88-89; Holahan et al. 1994, 32).

11. Coughlin et al. report that even accounting for funds obtained from special financing programs, state spending for medicaid increased 16 percent per year from 1988 to 1992 (1994b, 861).

12. The states included: Alabama, Arkansas, Florida, Georgia, Kentucky, Louisiana, Mississippi, North Carolina, South Carolina, Tennessee, West Virginia.

13. Only four states expanded their tax effort more than Massachusetts during the 1988-1991 era (Cromwell et al. 1994, 11-32).

14. By 1992, the following states had not implemented a special financing program: Alaska, Connecticut, Delaware, Idaho, Iowa, Nebraska, New Jersey, North Dakota, Oklahoma, Oregon, South Dakota, Virginia, and Wyoming (Cromwell et al., 1994, 11-32).

15. The term *public interest group* is comprised of the public officials and their lobby, "representing the political and administrative generalists" (Wright 1988, 281).

16. These organizations include the National Governors' Association (NGA), the National Conference of State Legislatures (NCSL), National League of Cities (NLC), U.S. Conference of Mayors (USCM), and National Association of Counties (NACO) (Wright 1988, 282).

17. Only six states had actually implemented such a program by 1990 (Coughlin et al. 1994, 92).

18. A Democratic HECC aide suggests that in 1991 President Bush and his Chief of Staff, former New Hampshire Governor John Sununu, intervened on New Hampshire's behalf to gain HCFA approval for the most extensive special financing program among all the states. Then-Governor Judd Gregg (R-NH), who was running for a Senate seat, faced a large budget shortfall in 1991, prior to the implementation of that state's medicaid financing scheme. Dan Morgan of *The Washington Post* attributes Gregg's 1992 Senate victory in part to the fact that he solved his state's fiscal problems without raising taxes (1993b).

19. Tremendous disagreement between Henry Waxman and OMB surfaced over the exact interpretation of the BEA, but ultimately, OMB won.

Conclusion

CHAPTER NINE

Implications of Policymaking for a Shared Program

Why is it that medicaid generates such fickle behavior among policymakers? Congress has vacillated in its affections toward that program since its conception. Likewise, the states both love and hate the program—soliciting its monetary favors, but repelling its mandatory requirements. However, since health care expenditures have grown higher and fiscal constraints have grown sharper at both levels of government, this instability has worsened. During the early 1980s both Congress and many states curtailed the medicaid program. Then, by the end of the same decade, both had dramatically enlarged its size and extent—the focus of this book. Now in the mid-1990s, with the states' apparent blessing, Congress is once again anticipating sharply limiting medicaid's scope.

Meanwhile, apart from one brief expansion and its immediate repeal, medicare has not enjoyed the periods of infatuation nor suffered the rejections of medicaid. Congress has treated medicare, especially its beneficiaries, more generously and more consistently. Under rising fiscal pressures, members of Congress have become increasingly interested in medicare as a source of cost-control, but have not demonstrated the same volatility toward it that they have toward medicaid. This chapter will first summarize what was learned about the politics of medicaid during the mid-1980s to early-90s, then discuss some of its implications for future medicaid policymaking.

SUMMARY OF FINDINGS

Congress

Conventional wisdom suggests and most of medicaid's history confirms that the medicaid program is easier for Congress to cut back than medicare, especially under conditions of economic strain. This view holds that, as a shared program targeted to the poor, medicaid lacks the political support of a national program, giving benefits by right, whose primary recipients are the elderly (Monypenny 1960, Morone 1991). But an aberration in this expected pattern of congressional behavior occurred from 1984 to 1990. During those years Congress repeatedly and extensively expanded medicaid while cutting back the medicare program. This study analyzed the circumstances that promoted this unusual expansion. They include the following:

Changes in the political, fiscal, and health care environments helped to propel the issue of medicaid expansions on to the congressional agenda. First, worsening problems of the health care sector stimulated the many secondary beneficiaries of medicaid to join forces and petition Congress for an increase in federal health care funding for the poor. Simultaneously, a change in the composition of Congress, to a more Democratic and liberal one, switched the priorities of that body from curtailing federal health care financing, to expanding it. But rising fiscal constraints heightened the importance of economic factors in choosing among various policy alternatives. Medicaid's federal-state shared financing made it the most politically and fiscally attractive alternative for expanding benefits because it enabled members of Congress to claim credit for providing benefits while shifting half of the cost to the states.

Although the issue of medicaid's expansion rose on the congressional agenda, the presence of significant obstacles—divided government; financial pressures; and opposition from the states, fiscal conservatives, and the president—might easily have derailed it. Without favorable changes in government institutions and a skillful and committed policy entrepreneur to exploit them, the scope of the extensions in medicaid would have been much more limited. Altered norms of federalism reduced congressional reticence about imposing intrusive and expensive mandates on the states during the 1980s. Furthermore, changes in the congressional budget process during that decade provided medicaid advocates with a unique legislative vehicle that helped them push medicaid through Congress with minimal opportunity for opposition or debate. And finally, Rep. Henry A. Waxman, strategically situated and highly skilled as a negotiator, engineered the strategy that enabled medicaid advocates to exploit the favorable political and institutional circumstances for extending medicaid.

States

During a period of great fiscal strain in the late 1980s and early 1990s, thirty nine states devised innovative financing techniques that allowed them to maximize their federal matching funds at no cost to themselves. Exploiting the open-ended, matched medicaid program allowed state policymakers to avoid more politically costly options to balance their budgets—raising taxes or cutting other programs. States' incentives to exploit this shared program were not new, but merely heightened by rising financial strain during the late 1980s. Their motivation to maximize medicaid was further augmented by the accumulation of federal mandates in that program, which had contributed significantly to the states' fiscal woes.

Although states have long possessed sufficient incentives, their ability to exploit this program has always been limited by the matching requirement. The emergence of a loophole in the medicaid law in the mid 1980s removed this obstacle. This change permitted states to expand their medicaid programs while shifting the entire cost of the extension to the federal government. As a result, states utilizing this option received a windfall in federal revenues. Many states failed to use that money to extend medicaid services or eligibility, but instead used it to balance their budgets.

The extent of the states' exploitation of medicaid was facilitated by several state-level as well as national-level factors. The increasingly professional staff and the strengthening of the institutions of interstate cooperation helped states create and disseminate critical information about how to take advantage of this loophole. However, had it not been for political and institutional factors at the national level, the states' ability to exploit the medicaid program would have been greatly limited.

The separation of powers and divided government at the national level permitted each branch to thwart the efforts of the other and created an atmosphere of distrust between the executive and legislative branches in the 1980s. HCFA recognized and attempted to halt the states' use of DSH financing schemes when they began, but because of HCFA's eagerness to gut the DSH program since the early 1980s, and because of HCFA's sluggishness in providing Congress clear data regarding the extent of the programs, Congress prevented HCFA from acting. This institutional arrangement of shared powers permitted the legislative branch to thwart the goals of the executive and blocked effective action against a raid on the federal treasury.

A liberal Congress, committed to extending medicaid and to permitting states great discretion in their financing strategies, blocked the efforts of a conservative administration more concerned with controlling medicaid expenditures. However, it appears that the White House, motivated by political concerns, also assisted key states in exploiting the DSH program before the full financial impact of such state behavior was known. Likewise, it was not only liberal members of Congress who helped states to maximize their cost-shifting strategies, but when HCFA regulations became inevitable, a number of conservative politicians also intervened on the behalf of their individual states to minimize its impact. Congress's local orientation, along with its liberalism was crucial. Because of this intervention, widespread use of these financing strategies spread throughout the states, and medicaid costs rose dramatically.

IMPLICATIONS FOR POLICYMAKING

This study reveals some troubling patterns and suggests some important lessons for current and future policymakers to heed. Given the likelihood that the two conditions that helped spawn these developments will endure, namely severe problems in the health care sector and fiscal constraints, it is important that we learn from the past. Some readers may draw lessons from this analysis regarding how to achieve national health insurance—through federal-state shared financing. Others may see it as justification for ending the open-ended feature of the medicaid program. At any event, this example has serious implications for health care policymaking for the future.

Sharing: Diffusion of Responsibility

Medicaid's shared funding and administration has affected its politics in a fundamental way: it diffuses responsibility. Structuring the program so that two levels of government make separate decisions regarding the program's scope and generosity permits neither to be responsible for the outcome. It allows each to make decisions that it would not make if it had sole responsibility for the fiscal and political consequences. At the federal level, this feature subjects medicaid to greater instability than a program that is fully federally funded. At the state level, it creates incentives to expand the medicaid program, rather than a state-only one, because of the state's ability to draw additional federal revenues.

Under conditions of fiscal strain, which have persisted since the early 1980s, shared programs such as medicaid provide policymakers advantages not offered by fully funded ones. Sharing makes it politically easier for Congress to cut or to expand that program than a fully federally funded one. Curtailing a shared program permits members to take credit for budgetary accomplishments, while leaving to the states the politically difficult decisions of how to implement the program reductions. When conservatives dominate the congressional agenda and cost control becomes a priority, shared programs such as medicaid are likely to be chosen for a disproportionate share of cuts, even though they do not deliver as great an economic savings as reducing fully federally funded ones.

However, as problems in the health care sector have worsened, a broad coalition has emerged to demand an increase in federal health care funding. Its strength varies over time, along with the partisan composition of Congress. When Democrats dominate the congressional agenda and the focus switches from cutting federal health care expenditures to expanding access, the shared medicaid program becomes the favorite choice. Given the economic restraints on policy choices, an enlargement in medicaid provides members the best opportunity to expand benefits while dispersing half the costs to the states.

Thus, the combined effects of fiscal constraints and worsening health care problems heighten the already unstable politics of medicaid. Under these conditions, which are likely to persist, congressional policymakers are prone to make greater cuts and larger extensions in medicaid than fully federally funded programs, such as medicare. Sharing permits them to do so without assuming full accountability for their actions. Although it has long been known that medicaid is more prone to program cutbacks than medicare, this analysis suggests it possesses a latent potential for expansion not previously recognized.

Since fiscal constraints and health care problems have worsened, the politics of medicaid have become even more unstable, following a cycle of curtailments (1981) and expansions (1984-1990). The enduring problems of the health care sector, especially problems of the uninsured and their impact on other health care actors, become more acute when federal funding is reduced. If a conservative Congress curtails the scope of medicaid, this is likely to stimulate the formation of a coalition seeking medicaid's enlargement, and, in the absence of major health care reform, the pendulum is likely to swing back once more, bringing expansion of that program back to the congressional agenda. Conservative policymakers should beware of the long term political impact of cutting back the shared medicaid program.

This diffusion in responsibility associated with shared programs also encourages states to expand those programs more than they would fully state-funded ones. The perverse incentives found in matched, open-ended grants are well-known (Beam 1980). Given the added fiscal pressures on states (e.g., federal mandates, anti-tax sentiment, balanced budget requirements), and the continued demand for increasing their health care expenditures (e.g., states as payers of last resort for the uninsured, Boren Amendment requirements), states look increasingly to the shared medicaid program as one of the most politically attractive sources of revenue. Given the rising level of sophistication among state government officials and their intergovernmental lobbying organizations, the ability of these officials to devise and implement complex and novel strategies to shift state expenses to the federal government has grown.

Recognizing the lack of accountability that is inherent in shared programs should alert policymakers at both levels to handle them with caution. Although the federal government is the 400 pound gorilla, in this relationship, able to impose costly mandates or damaging curtailments on the states against their will, they are far from defenseless creatures. They have found that the federal government can not continuously be watching and protecting every aspect of its programs from incremental assault. States are more creative and capable than ever of manipulating grants to accomplish their own will.

Incrementalism and Dispersion of Costs

Although national health reform was not on the congressional agenda during the 1980s, Congress went a long way toward implementing it. Henry Waxman took the lengthy approach to health care reform—year by year he added benefits for the nation's neediest. His patience, aided by the budget process that brought medicaid to the agenda, paid off. He also managed to disperse a large part of the costs to a non-voting entity—the states.

Medicare benefits were also expanded through an incremental approach, which Waxman also supported. So long as medicare benefits were added gradually, and the funding to cover them was widely dispersed, they aroused no controversy. However, when a dramatic extension in benefits was enacted in 1988, accompanied by an equally dramatic increase and concentration of costs to beneficiaries, the opposition was immediate and overwhelming. Few noticed that some of the extensions in benefits that were repealed in 1989 (e.g., hospice days, mammograms) were added in 1990, along with a sizable increase in the taxable wage base for HI, without so much as the bat of an eye. By dispersing the funding for medicare across a wider segment of the public, advocates for increased medicare benefits succeeded in inching their way toward their goal. Although the recent projections of medicare part A's early insolvency have forced policymakers to focus on ways to control expenditures, rather than expand benefits, this research suggests that incrementalism and the wide dispersion of medicare costs has been a politically effective formula for vastly increasing that program's revenues with minimal opposition.

Divided Government

Divided government at the national level played a significant role in permitting medicaid expenditures to accelerate during the early 1990s. Although its impact on state administration of federal grants requires further research, some lessons can be learned from this example. Without the separation of powers and divided government, accountability for medicaid's expenditures at the national level would have been clearer. State abuses of the DSH program would have been more readily detected and more responsibly controlled. Political incentives within each branch, and the conflict that existed in the 1980s between the branches, facilitated the states' raid on the federal treasury. HCFA would have issued appropriate regulations on the state use of DSH payments much earlier. This would have prevented $14 billion from being transferred from the federal to the state treasuries. It would almost certainly have resulted also in slower and less extensive implementation of the federal medicaid mandates, and greater state taxes or other state program curtailments.

This suggests that Congress was more amenable to the appeals of the states than its pattern of medicaid mandates suggests. Although it ignored state requests to stop enacting medicaid mandates in 1989 and 1990, it also extended the moratorium on HCFA regulations in those same years. This case illustrates more than mere divided government, but also the force of re-election goals at work.. Numerous members of both parties in Congress, both liberal and conservative, sought to find ways to assist their home states avoid costly new HCFA requirements in 1991. And, the White House supported their efforts. Sen. Rudman (R-NH), one of the architects of Gramm-Rudman-Hollings, was also one of the most active in assisting his home state to exploit the medicaid program. Even conservative members of Congress have a difficult time putting their money where their mouths are when the possibility exists to distribute concentrated benefits (especially to powerful interests) in their home states.

Lack of public scrutiny

The expansions in medicaid adopted by both levels of government were accomplished with little public scrutiny. By using the omnibus budget reconciliation bills as the primary congressional legislative vehicle, Congress limited debate and attention to these measures. However, their policy significance and their fiscal significance was great. Likewise at the state level, little public awareness of this policy existed outside the circle of state medicaid officials and health care providers, yet the impact on the federal budget was large. This tendency for policymakers to enact such expensive policies with little scrutiny suggests that their advocates feared they might not survive if they were subject to greater public attention.

However, keeping these issues out of the public eye hides the cost to society and helps to perpetuate a system of health care financing and delivery that is riddled with serious problems of efficiency and equity. One wonders, if the public were more aware of the perverse incentives and opportunities for cost-shifting that exist under the current shared public-private health care financing and delivery system—as medicaid illustrates—and if they knew who the winners and losers (taxpayers) are under such as system, would there not be greater demand to reform the health care system emerge?

Under conditions of fiscal strain, worsening problems in the health care sector, and a liberal Congress in the late 1980s, medicaid was transformed from the unpopular step-sister into the Cinderella of health care programs. For seven years it became the favorite target for expansion by both state and federal governments. However, a conservative mood now dominates Congress; midnight has struck; and Cinderella is once again subject to harsh treatment. Medicaid's shared funding, under circumstances of fiscal constraints, has served to intensify the volatility that has always plagued that program.

Major Medicaid Legislation 1965 to 1990

Year	Legislation and Provisions
1965	**Social Security Amendments of 1965 (P.L. 89-97)** • Established the medicaid program
1967	**Social Security Amendments of 1967 (P.L. 90-248)** • Limited eligibility for *medically needy* by establishing that the federal government would only provide matching funds to states where medicaid eligibility permitted the *medically needy* to earn no more than 150% of the state income standard for the ADFC assistance program. This limit would decrease to 133% in 1970. • Created Early, Periodic Screening, Diagnostic and Treatment (EPSDT) Program for children • Allowed states to purchase **Part B** medicare for *medically needy* elderly (not just welfare recipients) • Permitted states to add coverage for medicaid beneficiaries in intermediate care facilities • Required utilization review to guard against *unnecessary* utilization • Allowed states to add coverage for welfare beneficiaries in intermediate care facilities (ICFs)

Year	Legislation and Provisions
1969	**(P.L. 91-56)** • Permitted states to curtail *nonbasic* services • Required states desiring to curtail services to prove they were applying cost-control measures to medicaid administration and not increasing reimbursement to providers • Extended deadline for requiring states to establish comprehensive coverage from 1975 to 1977 • Allowed states to delay beginning steps towards comprehensiveness until July 1, 1971
1971	**Act of December 14, 1971 (P.L. 92-223)** • Permitted states to cover services for the *medically needy* provided in intermediate care facilities (ICFs) and ICFs for the mentally retarded
1972	**Social Security Amendments of 1972 (P.L. 92-603)** • Nationalized eligibility for welfare for the aged, blind, and disabled • Permitted states to continue using their previous standards for determining medicaid eligibility under section 209 (b) of this provision • Repealed 1902 (d) provision established in 1965 that required establishment of comprehensive medicaid coverage and maintenance of effort within states • Required coverage of family planning services • Permitted states to cover care for beneficiaries under 22 years old in psychiatric facilities (1965 legislation included care for those under 65 years) • Permitted states to extend coverage to include optometrists and chiropractors • Protected medicaid recipients from losing eligibility due to 20 % hike in social security benefits by extending eligibility for 4 months • Extended retroactive eligibility for 3 months for those found eligible (including the deceased)

Year	Legislation and Provisions
1972 (cont.)	• Established Professional Standards Review Organizations to monitor need and quality of care to recipients of medicare and medicaid • Established 1% reduction in federal share of AFDC payments for failure to comply with EPSDT requirements • Permitted states to charge nominal co-payments and deductibles for some medicaid recipients • Eliminated *statewideness and comparability* requirements with HEW approval so states could use pre-paid Health Maintenance Organizations (HMOs) where available
1973	**(P.L. 93-66)** • Maintained eligibility for 125,000 *essential persons* (spouses of SSI recipients who would otherwise lose it under new SSI regulations) • Extends protection for 9 months for medicaid recipients from losing eligibility due to 1972 hike in social security benefits
1976	**(P.L. 94-505)** • Established Office of Inspector General in DHEW to control fraud and abuse in medicare and medicaid
	(P.L. 94-566) • Preserved medicaid eligibility of recipients who become ineligible for cash SSI payments due to changes in the COLA in social security benefits • Protected married SSI recipients from a loss of medicaid benefits while the spouse was hospitalized
1977	**Rural Health Clinics Act (P.L. 95-201)** • Extends medicare and medicaid services to new health practitioners in rural clinics
	Medicare - Medicaid Anti-Fraud and Abuse Amendment of 1977 (P.L. 95-142) • Created Medicaid Fraud Control Units

Year	Legislation and Provisions
1980	**Mental Health Systems Act (P.L. 96-398)** • Required most states to create a computerized Medicaid Management Information System (MMIS) • Allowed waivers for home-and community-based care (only for those who would otherwise be cared for in an institution)
	Omnibus Reconciliation Act of 1980 (P.L. 96-499) • Boren Amendment repealed the requirement that states reimburse nursing home care on a *reasonable cost* basis • Extended coverage to include nurse-midwife services
	(P.L. 96-611) • Permitted states to restrict eligibility of children aged 18 to 21 under AFDC program to those in high school or vocational educational programs
1981	**Omnibus Budget Reconciliation Act of 1981 (P.L. 97-35)** • Extended Boren Amendment to inpatient hospital services • Reduced federal matching rates for 3 years for states whose payments exceeded certain targets: reductions of 3% in fiscal 1982, 4% in 1983, and 4.5% in 1984. • Tightened eligibility for AFDC, eliminating the inclusion of unborn children and 400,000 working poor families • Established waivers for freedom of choice and home and community-based services (only for those who would otherwise be cared for in an institution) • Eliminated special penalties for noncompliance with EPSDT requirements, making it easier for states not to comply • Gave states with *medically needy* coverage program greater authority to limit coverage • Allowed states to end medicaid coverage when a child reached 19 rather than 21 years of age • Increased states freedom to contract with HMOs • Repealed requirement to reimburse hospitals on basis of *reasonable cost* • Removed obligation to contract with PSROs, making it optional, for review of medicaid services

Year	Legislation and Provisions
1982	**Tax Equity and Fiscal Responsibility Act (TEFRA) of 1982** • Expanded eligibility to include home care for disabled children who would otherwise only be eligible as institutional recipients of SSI • Extended eligibility to pregnant women who would otherwise be eligible only after the birth of her child • Reduced federal payment to states whose error rates exceeded new federal standards • Permitted states to impose cost-sharing on certain recipients, except: children, pregnant women, and those institutionalized in long term care facilities with minimal income with certain restrictions on length of time and design of cost-sharing • Permitted states to impose liens on home of institutionalized persons under certain circumstances • Repealed the PSRO program, and instituted Peer Review Organizations (PROs)
1983	• **None**
1984	**Deficit Reduction Act (DEFRA) (P.L. 98-369)** • Mandated coverage of first-time pregnant women, pregnant women in two-parent families where the breadwinner was unemployed, and children (born after 10/1/83) up to age five in two-parent families • Permitted states to increase eligibility for AFDC and medicaid by raising the upper limit on family income from 150% to 185% of federal poverty level • Expanded eligibility for up to 15 months for employed persons losing AFDC due to changes in earned income disregards • Extended automatic eligibility to newborns of mothers receiving medicaid • Restricted eligibility to those who agree to assign to the states any right they had to other health benefits programs • Permitted states to enroll medicaid patients in state-qualified HMOs

Year	Legislation and Provisions
1984 (cont.)	• Raised assets SSI beneficiaries could have and still qualify • Relaxed requirements for certification by MDs that patients needed care in order to qualify for reimbursement in nursing facilities
	Child Support Enforcement Amendments of 1984 (P.L. 98-397) • Extends coverage for 4 months for children and caretakers who lose eligibility due to increased child support payments
1985	**Consolidated Omnibus Reconciliation Act (COBRA) of 1985 (P.L. 99-272)** • Extended medicaid coverage to pregnant women in two-parent, employed families who meet financial criteria for AFDC • Extended medicaid for 60 days post-partum to women who received medicaid during pregnancy • Permitted states to extend medicaid to certain foster care and adoptive children • Restored medicaid to certain widows and widowers losing SSI and medicaid due to changes in OASDI actuarial methods • Permitted states to provide additional benefits to pregnant women not normally covered for other medicaid beneficiaries • Permitted states to cover habilitation services to those discharged from long term care settings who participate in home- and community-based programs • Permitted states to cover home-and community-based services whose costs exceed estimated institutional care • Permitted states to cover hospice care • Permitted states to delete coverage of medically necessary, non-experimental organ transplants • Permitted states to extend case management services to some or all of their medicaid population • Disqualified certain persons shielding income and assets in *qualifying trusts*

Year	Legislation and Provisions
1986	**Omnibus Budget Reconciliation Act of 1986 (Public Law 99-509)** • Created new optional *categorically needy* group for aged and disabled with income below 100 percent of federal poverty line • Permitted states to cover pregnant women, and children under age 5 (phased in) with family incomes below 100% of federal poverty level. Permitted states to disregard assets. • Allowed states that extended eligibility to pregnant women and children to use medicaid to pay for medicare cost-sharing expenses for qualified Medicare beneficiaries (QMB) with incomes up to 100 percent of the federal poverty level • Allowed states to provide continuous coverage throughout pregnancy and post-partum regardless of changes in family income • Permitted states to extend temporary eligibility for pregnant women who are initially presumed to be eligible for full coverage • Required medicaid coverage of the disabled enrolled in SSI that lose SSI due to earnings, who need medicaid to continue working, and whose earnings do not replace benefits lost • Eliminated coverage of illegal aliens • Permitted states to extend community-based care to those with AIDS and those with mental illness who would otherwise be institutionalized • Permitted coverage of home care for the ventilator-dependent • Required external audits of HMOs participating in medicaid • Clarifies that state must make medicaid available to the homeless • Held states harmless as a result of the change from biennial to annual calculation of state matching funds

Year	Legislation and Provisions
	Immigration Reform and Control Act (P.L. 99-473) • Extended medicaid to otherwise eligible temporary resident aliens who are pregnant, children, or those with emergency medical conditions, elderly or disabled
1987	**Omnibus Budget Reconciliation Act of 1987 (P.L. 100-203)** • Permitted states to cover all pregnant women and infants with incomes under 185% of the federal poverty level • Allowed immediate expansion of OBRA 1986 coverage up to 100% of poverty line for children up to age 5 • Allowed coverage for children aged 5-7, up to state AFDC levels (phased in) • Allowed coverage for children below 9 years of age up to 100% of federal poverty level (phased in) • Allowed home- and community-based services to the elderly who would otherwise need to be institutionalization • Broadly reformed standards for certifying and measuring the performance of long term care facilities • Required states to implement 1986 regulations to make additional payments to Disproportionate Share Hospitals • Allowed states to pay the costs of health services delivered by clinics to the homeless
1988	**Medicare Catastrophic Coverage Act of 1988 (P.L. 100-360)** • Made mandatory the OBRA 1986 option of providing medicaid coverage for pregnant women and infants with incomes up to 100% of the federal poverty level (phased in) • Made mandatory the OBRA 1986 option of states to pay for medicare cost-sharing expenses of QMBs with incomes up to 100% of the federal poverty level (phased in) • Established higher minimum levels of protected income and assets for spouses of institutionalized individuals • Protected medicaid eligibility of AFDC recipients and the *medically needy* by prohibiting states from reducing AFDC payments below May 1988 levels

Year	Legislation and Provisions
1988 (cont.)	• Clarified state obligation to pay for education-related services to disabled children • Permitted states to establish more generous medicaid eligibility standards and methods for non-cash assistance applicants • Established moratorium preventing HHS from publishing final regulations to limit the state's ability to use donated funds through 12/31/89
	Family Support Act of 1988 (P.L. 100-485) • Increased required period of medicaid coverage if AFDC cash assistance is lost due to earnings • Required medicaid coverage for two-parent unemployed families if otherwise eligible. • Liberalized rules for treatment of earned income for AFDC and medicaid purposes
1989	**Omnibus Budget Reconciliation Act of 1989 (P.L. 101-239)** • Required states to extend coverage to pregnant women, infants, and children up to 6 years of age, if income is below 133% of the federal poverty level • Required states to provide care needed to correct problems identified in children under the EPSDT program, even if not otherwise covered under state medicaid plan and required more frequent periodic screenings under the EPSDT program when medical problems are suspected • Required states to cover pediatric nurse practitioner services to the extent such services are permitted by state law • Required that state reimbursement of medicaid providers be *sufficient* to ensure that services are as adequate for medicaid recipients as they would be for the general public and to provide documentation that payment levels for pediatric and obstetrical services meet this requirement

Year	Legislation and Provisions
1989 (cont.	• Required states to coordinate their medicaid programs with that of the food program for women, infants and children (WIC) • Required states to pay medicare Part A premiums for certain qualified working disabled • Required states to include Federally Qualified Health Centers as medicaid providers and to reimburse them 100% of reasonable costs • Extended until 12/31/90 moratorium preventing HHS from publishing final regulations to limit the state's ability to use donated funds
1990	**Omnibus Budget Reconciliation Act of 1990 (P.L. 101-508)** • Required states to provide coverage to children up to age 18, if income is below 100% of the federal poverty level (phased in) • Required states to provide coverage to women throughout the post-partum period that was made optional under OBRA 1986 • Extended the period of presumptive eligibility for pregnant women before a written medicaid application is required • Required states to receive and process applications for pregnant women and children at convenient outreach sites • Required states to offer continuous eligibility to infants if they were born to a medicaid-eligible mother *and* remain in the mother's household • Extended the MCCA *qualified Medicare beneficiary* (QMB) provision to those with incomes below 120% of the federal poverty level (phased in) • Allowed states to develop home- and community-based programs for the disabled and mentally retarded. • Permitted certain states to liberalize *medically needy* income standard for a single person

Year	Legislation and Provisions
1990 (cont.)	• Required states to pay health insurance premiums where cost effective and pay other cost-sharing for beneficiaries who are otherwise eligible for private insurance • Required states to establish drug rebate program meeting federal standards or lose matching funds for drugs • Required state to impose prior authorization regulations for certain drugs • Extended through 12/31/91 the moratorium preventing HHS from publishing final regulations to limit the state's ability to use donated funds

Sources: *Congress and the Nation,* Vols. 2-8; *Social Security Bulletin, Annual Statistical Supplement,* 1993.

Major Medicare Legislation 1965 to 1990

Year	Legislation and Provisions
1965	**Social Security Amendments of 1965 (P.L. 89-97)** • Established the medicare program • Established that the federal government would only provide matching funds to states where medicaid eligibility permitted the *medically needy* to earn no more than 150% of the state income standard for the ADFC assistance program. This limit would decrease to 133% in 1970. • Established **Part B** monthly premiums to pay 1/2 of **Part B** costs; deductible set at $10 per month • Established Hospital Insurance (HI) tax on the self-employed, employees, and employers on income up to $6,600 and a schedule of increases up to a maximum rate of .8% by the year 1987 • Established deductible for **Part A** at $40
1966	**(P.L. 89-384)** • Extended deadline for signing up for **Part B** • Permitted *for-profit* nursing homes a profit of 7.5% on services to medicare patients
1967	**Social Security Amendments of 1967 (P.L. 90-248)** • Added 60 days *lifetime reserve* for in-patient services • Added ancillary hospital services and extended care facility services

Year	Legislation and Provisions
1967 (cont.)	• Added out-patient physical therapy, diagnostic x-rays, and purchase of durable medical equipment • Permitted annual enrollment in **Part B** • Allowed states to purchase **Part B** for the *medically needy* (not just welfare recipients) • Increased the taxable wage base for **Part A** from $6,600 to $7,800 and phased in and increase in the contribution rate beginning 1/68 to a total of 5.9% (OASDI and HI) in 1987
1968	**(P.L. 90-)** • Increased deductible for **Part A** in-patient care
1972	**Social Security Amendments of 1972 (P.L. 92-603)** • Extended eligibility to 1.7 million disabled under age 65 and to those with End Stage Renal Disease • Extended benefits to cover services of residents of podiatry training, outpatient physical therapy, chiropractic, speech pathology, and some optometry services. • Limited the premium rate that beneficiaries paid for medicare **Part B** to the rate of increase in cash benefits • Phased in an increase in the OASDHI tax rate and taxable income to 5.85 % and $12,000 in 1974 over previous law • Established Professional Standards Review Organizations (PSROs) to monitor need and quality of care to recipients of medicare and medicaid. • Enabled beneficiaries to enroll in approved HMOs • Allowed those over 65 years, enrolled in **Part B** who is not otherwise entitled to **Part A** benefits, to pay a monthly premium to participate in **Part A**
1973	**(P.L. 93-233)** • Increased Social Security payroll tax wage base to $13,200 from $12,600 beginning 1/1/74 • Altered tax rates among Social Security trust funds, increasing OASDI by 0.1% while decreasing HI by 0.1%
1975	**(P.L. 94-182)** • Delayed deadline for setting up PSROs • Enabled some states to place PSROs under state medical society control

Year	Legislation and Provisions
1976	**(P.L. 94-368)** • Permanently barred any decrease in federal reimbursement rates to MD below 1975 levels, delayed increases in reimbursement to MD and hospitals
	(P.L. 94-505) • Established Office of Inspector General in DHEW to control frauds and abuse in medicare and medicaid
1977	**Medicare - Medicaid Anti-Fraud and Abuse Amendment of 1977 (P.L. 95-142)** • Created Medicare and Medicaid Fraud Control Units and upgraded penalties
	Rural Health Clinics Act (P.L. 95-201) • Extended medicare and medicaid coverage to new health practitioners in rural clinics
1980	**Omnibus Reconciliation Act of 1980 (P.L. 96-499)** • Extended coverage to disabled who lost cash benefits due to substantial gainful employment • Eliminated second waiting period for disabled if entitled again within 5 years • Removed limits on number of home health visits • Extended outpatient benefits • Authorized payments without the usual cost-sharing requirement for outpatient alcohol treatment, diagnostic test, and certain surgical procedures • Increased ceiling on outpatient physical therapy • Repealed limits on re-enrollment in **Part B**
1981	**Omnibus Budget Reconciliation Act of 1981 (P.L. 97-35)** • Increased the deductible for **Part A** and **Part B** services moderately • Eliminated carryover of incurred expenses from previous year for meeting **Part B** deductible • Tightened reimbursement limits for hospital operating costs • Limited open enrollment period from 12 to 2 months per year

Year	Legislation and Provisions
1982	**Tax Equity and Fiscal Responsibility Act of 1982 (P.L. 97-248)** • Extended **Part A** coverage to include hospice care • Recognized HMOs as providers of care for **Part A** • Established limits on annual rate of increase for total hospital costs per discharge. • Made certain federal employees eligible for medicare and required them to pay HI tax • Increased the share the elderly would otherwise pay for **Part B** by setting the premium costs at one-fourth the cost of the program for elderly beneficiaries
1983	**Social Security Amendments of 1983 (P.L. 98-21)** • Established prospective payment scheme based upon DRGs for inpatient care under **Part A** to be phased in over three years • Established Peer Review Organizations (PROs), to replace PSROs, charge with overseeing quality of care and preventing unnecessary hospitalization • Made employees of non-profit organizations eligible for medicare, requiring them to pay HI tax • Recognized HMOs as providers of care for **Part B**
1984	**Deficit Reduction Act (DEFRA) 1984 (P.L. 98—369)** • Imposed a temporary freeze on physician fees • Reduced payment amount for durable medical equipment provided by home health agencies • Extended outpatient services covered under **Part B** • Reestablished the provisions that sets the premium for **Part B** at one-fourth the cost of the program for elderly beneficiaries for two years • Limits the increase in **Part B** premium to the increase in the COLA for social security
1985	**Consolidated Omnibus Reconciliation Act of 1985 (COBRA) (P.L. 99-272)** • Made eligibility in medicare **Part A** mandatory for virtually all state and local employees hired after 12/31/85 and voluntary for those hired earlier

Year	Legislation and Provisions
1985 (cont.)	• Extended eligibility for **Part A** to anyone 65 years or older who pays the monthly premium for **Part A** • Expanded **Part A** benefits to include liver transplants • Limited the increase in **Part B** premiums through 1988 to that of the 1986 level • Made permanent coverage and increases reimbursement rates for hospice care • Instituted numerous adjustments in reimbursements to hospitals designed to save money and increase equity among various types of facilities • Imposed penalties on hospitals "dumping" poor patients to other facilities • Extended by one year the phasing in of prospective payment • Extended existing freeze on MD reimbursement until 12/31/86
1986	**Omnibus Reconciliation Act of 1987 (P.L. 99-509)** • Capped 1987 **Part A** deductible at $520, ($52 below what it would have been),and slowed the rate of growth for further increases • Instituted a number of changes in reimbursements to hospitals, including: increasing DRG payment, changing the way of determining DRG rate, allowing rural hospitals to qualify for DSH payments, altering reimbursement for outpatient surgery • Prohibited hospitals, HMOs, and CMPs from providing financial incentives to MD for reducing services to medicare beneficiaries • Granted 3.2% increase in MD reimbursement and made permanent a differential between participating and non participating MD • Reduced reimbursement for certain procedures

Year	Legislation and Provisions
1986 (cont.)	• Extended **Part A and B** coverage of certain services performed by occupational therapist, physician services, nurse anesthetists, optometrists • Extended **Part B** surgical coverage to include those performed in outpatient settings
1987	• **Budget Reconciliation Act of 1988 (P.L. 100-203)** • Established numerous provisions designed to reduce reimbursements overall while increasing equity for providers of all sorts • Permitted previously disabled individuals to resume coverage without 2 year waiting period • Increased coverage and reimbursement for mental health services • Restricted eligibility for home health care • Extended **Part B** coverage to non-physician providers, including: nurse-midwives, clinical psychologists, physician assistants • Continued (through 1989) to require **Part B** premiums to cover 25% of that program's costs, but held beneficiaries harmless through blocking increases in premiums that exceeded the COLA in OASDI cash benefits
1988	**Medicare Catastrophic Coverage Act (MCCA) of 1988 (P.L. 100-360)** • Extended coverage to outpatient drugs • Extended a number of benefits to cover catastrophic medical expenses, limiting the financial risk to beneficiaries • Increased **Part B** premium for all beneficiaries, and established an income-related premium for **Part A**
1989	**Medicare Catastrophic Coverage Repeal Act (MCCRA) of 1989 (P.L. 101-234)** • Repealed medicare catastrophic benefits of MCCA • Canceled changes in **Part A** and **Part B** premiums

Year	Legislation and Provisions
	Omnibus Reconciliation Act of 1989 (OBRA) **(P.L. 101-239)** • Revised medicare physician payment system—Resource Based Relative Value Scale (RBRVS)to be phased in over 5 years • Limited amount physicians may charge patients over and above medicare reimbursement' • Extended through 1990 a provision that **Part B** premiums cover 25% of the program's costs • Instituted numerous reductions in payments for various procedures and made adjustments designed to reduce expenditures • Required GAO conduct a number of studies related to various matters, including standards to determine medical necessity, administrative costs of medicare requirements for insurers and providers, effect of ownership of facilities on quality of care and utilization by patients. • Expanded **Part B** coverage of non-physician health care providers in various settings • Extended **Part B** coverage to include Pap smears • Instituted a number of reimbursement changes for **Part A** to continue to reduce expenditures and address concerns of specific types of hospitals to correct perceived inequities • Barred nursing homes from charging medicare patients more than the medicare-approved amount • Created a new agency to conduct research related to effectiveness and appropriateness of medical care—AHCPR • Eliminated **Part B** limits on mental health services

Year	Legislation and Provisions
1990	• **Omnibus Reconciliation Act of 1990 (OBRA) (P.L. 101-508)** • Raised from $75 to $100 the deductible for **Part B** • Continued requiring that beneficiaries of **Part B** pay 25% of the cost of that program through their premiums. Set the rates in advance through 1995, rather than allowing them to float. • Increased taxable income for HI tax to $125,000 and established a formula for automatic increases in the wage base as incomes rise • Boosted payments to inner city and rural hospitals • Required hospitals to inform patients about "living wills" • Reduced payments for 244 procedures deemed to be overpaid by medicare • Included numerous reimbursement provisions designed to tighten payments for hospitals, physicians, laboratories, medical equipment • Extended length of hospice benefits beyond 210 days (had been in the 1988 MCCA which was repealed in 1989) • Expanded coverage to include mammograms, injectable drugs for osteoporosis, Erythropoietin for ESRD • Loosened requirements on HMOs to be able to offer financial incentives to MD in order to decrease the use of patient services

Sources: *Congress and the Nation,* Vols 2-8; *Annual Statistical Supplement to the Social Security Bulletin,* 1993.

References

Advisory Commission on Intergovernmental Relations. 1992. *Significant Features of Fiscal Federalism*. Document M-180. Washington: Government Printing Office, February.

Advisory Commission on Intergovernmental Relations. 1984. *Regulatory Federalism: Policy, Process, Impact and Reform*. Document A-95. Washington: Government Printing Office, February.

Anderson, Gerard and William Scanlon. 1993. "Medicaid Payment Policy and the Boren Amendment." In *Medicaid Financing Crisis: Balancing , Responsibilities, Priorities, and Dollars*, ed. Diane Rowland, Judith Feder, Alina Salganicoff. San Francisco: American Association for the Advancement of Science.

Anton, Thomas J. 1989. *American Federalism and Public Policy: How the System Works*. Philadelphia, PA: Temple University.

Arnold, R. Douglas. 1990. *The Logic of Congressional Action*. New Haven, Conn.: Yale University.

Ball, Robert M. 1995. "Perspectives on Medicare." *Health Affairs* 14(4): 62–88.

Bardach, E. 1977. *The Implementation Game*. Cambridge, Mass.: Massachussetts Institute of Technology.

Barone, Michael and Grant Ujifusa. 1986. *Almanac of American Politics*. Washington, D.C.: National Journal.

Barone, Michael, Grant Ujifusa, and Douglas Matthews. 1980. *Almanac of American Politics*. Washington, D.C.: National Journal.

Barrilleaux, Charles J. and Mark E. Miller. 1992. "Decisions without Consequences: Cost Control and Access in State Medicaid Programs." *Journal of Health Politics, Policy and Law* 17(1): 97–118.

Beer, Samuel. 1977. "Political Overload and Federalism." *Polity* 10: 5–17.

Beam, David. 1980. "Economic Theory as Policy Prescription: Pessimistic Findings on Optimizing Grants." In *Why Policies Succeed or Fail*, ed. Helen M. Ingram and Dean E. Mann. Beverly Hills, Calif.: Sage.

Bovbjerg, Randall R. and John Holahan. 1982. *Medicaid in the Reagan Era: Federal Policy and State Choices*. Washington, D.C.:The Urban Institute.

Brown, Lawrence D. 1983. *New Policies, New Politics: Government's Response to Government's Growth. Washington*, D.C.: The Brookings Institution.

Buck, Jeffrey A. and John Klemm. 1992. "Recent Trends in Medicaid Expenditures" *Health Care Financing Review* (Annual Supplement): 217–283.

Burke, Marybeth. 1991. "Medicaid Expansion Creates New Dilemma For State Programs." *Hospitals* (65)3: 34–36.

Chubb, John E. 1995. "The Political Economy of Federalism." *American Political Science Review* 79:994–1015.

Claiborne, William. 1992. "Health Costs Squeeze State Budgets: Report Shows Revenue Growth Lags Behind Medicaid Increases," *Washington Post,* 29 October.

Claiborne, William. 1993."States Demand an Explanation: Federal Lawmakers Summoned To Justify Unfunded Mandates," *Washington Post*, 5 July.

Cohen, Sally S. 1991. "The Politics of Medicaid: 1980–1989." *Nursing Outlook.* 38:229–233.

Cohodes, Donald R. "America: The Home of the Free, the Land of the Uninsured." *Inquiry* 23:227–235.

Congressional Budget Office. 1991. *Universal Health Insurance Coverage Using Medicare's Payment Rates.* Washington, D.C.: U. S. Government Printing Office, December.

Congressional Budget Office.1992. *Factors Contributing to the Growth of the Medicaid Program*. Staff Memorandum. May.

Congressional Quarterly Almanac. 1987. "Reconciliation Bill Raises Taxes, Cuts Spending." 42:615–627.

———, 1986. "The O'Neill Era Comes to an End in the House." 42: 29–35.

Congress and the Nation, 1965–1968, Vol.2. Washington, D.C.: Congressional Quarterly.

———, *1969–1972,* Vol. 3. Washington, D.C.: Congressional Quarterly.

———, *1973–1976,* Vol. 4. Washington, D.C.: Congressional Quarterly.

——— *1977–1980,* Vol. 5. Washington, D.C.: Congressional Quarterly.

———, *1981–1984,* Vol. 6. Washington, D.C.: Congressional Quarterly.

———, *1985–1988,* Vol. 7. Washington, D.C.: Congressional Quarterly.

———, *1989–1992*, Vol. 8. Washington, D.C.: Congressional Quarterly.

Congressional Research Service.1992. *Medicaid: Recent Trends in Beneficiaries and Spending*. Document no. LTR92–648. Washington: Library of Congress.

Coughlin, Teresa A., Leighton Ku, and John Holahan. 1994a. *Medicaid Since 1980: Costs, Coverage, and the Shifting Alliance Between the Federal Government and the States*. Washington, D.C.: Urban Institute.

Coughlin, Teresa A., Leighton Ku, John Holahan, David Heslam, and Colan Winterbottom. 1994b. "State Responses to Medicaid Spending Crisis: 1988 to 1992." *Journal of Health Politics, Policy and Law* 19(4): 837–864.

Cromwell, Jerry, Ann Boulis, Killard W. Amanche, Carol Ammering, and William J. Bartosch. 1994. *Examining The Medicaid Fiscal Crisis*. Massachuesetts:Center for Health Economics Research, October.

Davidson, Roger H. 1989. "The Senate: If Everybody Leads, Who Follows?" In *Congress Reconsidered*, 4th ed., ed. Lawrence C. Dodd and Bruce I. Oppenheimer. Washington D.C.: Congressional Quarterly.

Davidson, Roger H. 1992. *The Postreform Congress*. New York: St. Martin's.

Davidson, Roger H. and Walter J. Oleszek.1994. *Congress and Its Members*. 4th ed. Washington D.C.: Congressional Quarterly.

Deignan, Kathy. 1995. Telephone conversation with the author, 10 October.

Demokovich, Linda E. 1984. " For Poor and Elderly, Congress's Cuts In Health Budgets Have Silver Lining." *National Journal* 16: 1309–11.

Department of Political Science, Northeastern University. 1992. *Insuring American Health for the Year 2000*. Boston, Mass.: Northeastern University, June.

Derthick, Martha. 1970. *The Influence of Federal Grants: Public Assistance in Massachusetts*. Cambridge, Mass.: Harvard University.

———. 1975. *Uncontrollable Spending For Social Services Grants*. Washington D.C.: The Brookings Institution.

———. 1987. "American Federalism: Madison's Middle Ground in 1980's." *Public Administration Review* 47(1): 66–74.

———. 1992. "Federal Government Mandates: Why the States Are Complaining." *The Brookings Review* 4(10): 50–53.

———. 1996. "Crossing Thresholds: Federalism in the 1960s." *Journal of Policy History,* forthcoming.

Dionne, Jr. E.J. 1987. "Children Emerge as Issue for Democrats." *New York Times,* 27 September.

Durman, Gene. 1981. *The Study of Federal Grants-In-Aid in Health and Social Services: the Implications of the Fiscal Constraints Study.* Project Report 1389–18. Washington, D.C.: The Urban Institute.

Economic Report of the President. 1994. U.S. Government Printing Office. February.

Etheredge, Lynn. 1986. "Ethics and the New Insurance Market." *Inquiry* 23: 308–15.

Farley, Pamela J. 1985. "Who Are The Uninsured?" *Milbank Memorial Fund Quarterly* 63:476–508.

Farney, Dennis and Joe Davidson, 1989. "States Grow Restive About Picking Up the Tab For Social Programs Mandated By Washington," *Wall Street Journal*, September 14.

Feder, Judith M. 1991. "Health Care of the Disadvantaged: The Elderly" In *Health Policy and the Disadvantaged,* ed. Lawrence Brown. Durham, N.C.:Duke University.

Feder, Judith M. and Diane Rowland. 1992, "Government. " *Journal of the American Medical Association* 268(3):362–364.

Feldstein, Paul J. 1988. *The Politics of Health Legislation: An Economic Perspective.* Ann Arbor, MI: Health Administration.

Ferejohn, John A. 1991. "Changes in Welfare Policy in the 1980s" in *Politics and Economics of the Eighties*, ed. Alberto Alsina and Geoffrey Carliner. Chicago: University of Chicago.

Ferejohn, John and Keith Kriehbiel. 1987. "The Budget Process and the Size of the Budget." *American Journal of Political Science* 31:296–320.

Fessler, James F. and Donald F. Kettl. 1991. *The Politics of the Administrative Process.* Chatham, NJ, Chatham House.

Fraser, Irene. 1991. "Health Policy and Access to Care" in *Health Politics and Policy,* 2d ed., ed. Theodor J. Litman and Leonard S. Robins. New York: Delmar.

Fossett, James W. and James H. Wyckoff. 1992. "Has Medicaid Growth Crowded Out State Education Spending?" Presented to Department of Public Administration and Policy at the APPAM Research Conference, Denver, Colorado, November.

Fossett, James W. et al. 1992. "Medicaid and Access to Child Health Care in Chicago." *Journal of Health Policy Politics and Law* 17(2): 273–98.

Fuchs, Beth C. and John F. Hoadley. 1987. "Reflections from Inside the Beltway: How Congress and the President Grapple with Health Policy." *P.S. Political Science* 20:212-220.

General Accounting Office. 1990. *The Budget Deficit: Outlook, Implications, and Choices.* Washington, D.C.: Government Printing Office.

General Accounting Office. 1991. *Medicaid Expansions: Coverage Improves but State Fiscal Problems Jeopardize Continued Progress.* General Accounting Office/ HRD-91–78. June.

Gilmour, John B. 1990. *Reconcilable Differences*: Congress, *The Budget Process, and the Deficit.* Berkely: University of California.

Gold, Steven D. 1992. "The Federal Role in State Fiscal Stress." *Publius,* 34:33–47.

———. 1993a. "Passing The Buck." *State Legislatures* 19(1):36–38.

———.1993b. "The State Budget Context: How Medicaid Fits In." In *Medicaid Financing Crisis: Balancing , Responsibilities, Priorities, and Dollars*, ed. Diane Rowland, Judith Feder, Alina Salganicoff. San Francisco: American Association for the Advancement of Science.

Gramlich, Edward M. 1990. "The Economics of Fiscal Federalism and Its Reform." In *The Changing Face of Fiscal Federalism, ed.* Thomas R. Swartz and John E. Peck. Armonk, N.Y.: M.E. Sharpe, Inc.

Grogan, Colleen. 1993. "Federalism and Health Care Reform." *American Behavioral Scientist* 36:741–759.

Haas, Lawrence J. 1991. "Creative Financing." *National Journal.* 29: 1804–1807.

Hahm, Sung Deuk et al. 1992. "The Influence of the Gramm-Rudman-Hollings Act on Federal Budgetary Outcomes, 1986–1989." *Journal of Policy Analysis and Management* 11:207–234.

Hall, William K. 1989. *The New Institutions of Federalism.* New York: Peter Lang.

Hart, Henry. 1955. "The Relationship between States and Federal Law" in *Federalism: Mature and Emergent, ed.* Arthur W. McMahon. New York: Doubleday.

Hinds, Michael deCourcy. 1990. "The Governors Talk About Taxing and Spending," *New York Times,* 28 October.

Holahan, John et al. 1992. *States' Response to Medicaid Financing Crisis.* Washington, D.C.: Urban Institute. December.

Holahan, John, et al. 1993. "Understanding the Recent Growth in Medicaid Spending," In *Medicaid Financing Crisis: Balancing, Responsibility, Priorities, and Dollars,.* ed. Diane Rowland, Judith Feder, Alina Salganicoff. San Francisco: American Association for the Advancement of Science.

Holahan, John F. and Joel W.Cohen. 1986. *Medicaid: The Trade-off Between Cost Containment and Access to Care.* Washington, D.C.: The Urban Institute Press.

Hook, Janet. 1985. "House Energy Committee OKs Medicare, Medicaid Changes." *Congressional Quarterly Weely Review* 43:1554

———. 1985. "Senate, House at Odds Over Health Spending." *Congressional Quarterly Weekly Review* 43:1056.

Kimball, Merit C. 1991. "States Blast Bush's Provider Tax Ban." *HealthWeek,* September 23.

Kingdon, John W. 1984. *Agendas, Alternatives and Public Policies.* Toronto: Little, Brown and Company.

Kinney, Eleanor D. 1991. "Rule and Policy Making for the Medicaid Program: A Challenge to Federalism." *Ohio State Law Journal* 51: 877–911.

Kirschten, Dick. 1989. "Don't Bill Us." *National Journal* 21:3044–3047.

Koch, Edward I. 1980. "The Mandate Millstone." *Public Interest Journal* 61 (Fall):42–57.

Kogan, Richard. 1995. Telephone conversation with the author. 12 October.

Kosterlitz, Julie. 1988. "Not Just Kid Stuff." *The National Journal* 20: 2934–39.

———. 1989. "Watch Out for Waxman." *The National Journal* 21: 577–581.

Kovner, Anthony R. 1995. *Health Care Delivery In The United States.* 5th ed. New York.: Springer.

Krane, Dale. 1993. "State Efforts to Influence Federal Policy." In *Welfare System Reform: Coordinating Federal, State, and Local Public Assistance Programs,* ed. Edward T. Jennings and Neal S. Zank. Wesport, CN: Greeenwood Press.

Ku, Leighton and Teresa A.Coughlin. 1995. "Medicaid Disproportionate Share and Other Special Financing Programs." *Health Care Financing Review* 16(3): 27–54.

Letsch, Suzanne W., Helen C. Lazenby, Katherine R. Levit, Cathy A. Cowan. 1992. "National Health Expenditures, 1991." *Health Care Financing Review* 14(2): 1–30.

Levit, Katherine R. and Cathy A. Cowan.1990."The Burden of Health Care Costs: Business, Households, and Governments." *Health Care Financing Review* 12(2): Table 7.

Levit, Katherine R., Gry L. Olin, Suzanne W. Letsch. 1992. "Ámerican's Health Insurance Coverage, 1980–1991." *Health Care Financing Review* 14(1): 31–58.

Long, Stephen H. 1993. "Causes of Soaring Medicaid Spending, 1988–1991." In *Medicaid Financing Crisis: Balancing Responsibilities, Priorities, and Dollars,* ed. Diane Rowland, Judith Feder, Alina Salganicoff. San Franscisco: American Association for the Advancement of Science.

Mandel, Michael J. and Christopher Farrell. 1991. "The Sad State of the States." *Business Week,* 22 April: 24–26.

Marchasin, Sidney. 1991. "Cost Shifting: How One Hospital Does It," *Wall Street Journal,* 9 November.

Marmor, Theodore M. 1983. Introduction to *Political Analysis and American Medical Care.* Cambridge, Mass.: Cambridge University.

Martin, James.1995. Telephone conversation with the author, 10 October.

Merlis, Mark. 1991. *Medicaid: Provider Donations and Provider Specific Taxes Report for Congress.* No. 91–722 EPW. Congressional Research Service, Library of Congress. October 2.

Merrill, Teri. 1987. "HCFA Challenges State's Retention of Medicaid Funds." *Hospitals,* 20 May, 26.

Miller, Victor J. 1993. "State Medicaid Expansion in the Early 1990s." In *Medicaid Financing Crisis: Balancing Responsibilities, Priorities, and Dollars,* ed. Diane Rowland, Judith Feder, and Alina Salganicoff, San Francisco: American Association for the Advancement of Science.

Monypenny, Phillip. 1960. "Federal Grants-in-Aid to State Governments: A Political Analysis." *National Tax Journal* 13:1–16.

Moon, Marilyn. 1993. *Medicare Now and in the Future.* Washington D.C.: Urban Institute.

Morgan, Dan. 1993a. "Medicaid Loopholes Closing for Strapped States." *Washington Post,* 7 February.

———. 1993b. "Medicaid Windfall Cut State Deficits." *Washington Post,* 28 February.

———. 1993c. "States' Medicaid Prognosis Improves." *Washington Post,* 21 April.

———. 1994a. "Medicaid Grows Into 'Budget Time Bomb:' How Health Program for the Poor Expanded Into Entitlement With Few Cost Controls." *Washington Post,* 30 January.

———. 1994b. "Small Provision Turns Into a Golden Goose." *Washington Post,* 31 January.

———. 1994c. "Medicaid Windfall Cut State Deficits: N.H., Others Used Loopholes While Bloating U.S. Budget," *Washington Post,* 28 February.

Morone, James A. 1991. "The Politics of Health Care Reform." In *Health Politics and Policy*. 2d ed., ed. Theodor J. Litman, and Leonard S. Robins. New York: Delmar.

Morris, Dwight. 1992. *Handbook of Campaign Spending*. Washington, D.C.: Congressional Quarterly.

National Center for Health Services Research. 1989. "Health Insurance Coverage of Retired Persons." Research Findings 2, *National Medical Expenditure Survey*. Washington, D.C.: Department of Health and Human Services.

Nathan, Richard P. 1993. "The Role of the States in American Federalism" *In the State of the States*. 2d ed., ed. Carl van Horn. Washington D.C.: Congressional Quarterly.

Neckerman, Kathryn M., Robert Aponte, and William Julius Wilson. 1988. "Family Structure, Black Unemployment, and American Social Policy." In *The Politics Of Social Policy in the United States*, ed. Margaret Weir, Ann Shola Orloff, and Theda Skocpol. Princeton, NJ.:Princeton University.

Oberg, Charles and Cynthia Longseth Polich. 1988. "Medicaid." *Health Affairs* 7(3):83–96.

Oleszek, Walter J. 1996, *Congressional Procedures and the Policy Process*. 4th ed. Washignton, D.C.: Congressional Quarterly.

Palazzolo, Daniel J. 1992. "From Decentralization to Centralization: Members' Changing Expectations for House Leaders."In *The Postreform Congress*, ed. Roger H. Davidson. New York: St. Martin's.

Patterson, James T. 1981. *America's Struggle Against Poverty, 1900–1980*. Cambridge, Mass.:Harvard University.

Pear, Robert. 1990. "Deficit or No Deficit, Unlikely Allies Bring About Expansion in Medicaid." *New York Times,* 4 November.

Peirce, Neal R. 1991. "State Budget Disasters: Any Way Out?" *National Journal* 23:1008.

Peterson, Paul E., Barry G. Rabe, Kenneth K. Wong. 1986. *When Federalism Works*. Washington D.C.: The Brookings Institution.

Plattner, Andy. 1983. "No Better Issues Committee: Scrappy House Energy Panel Provides High Pressure Arena For Wrangling Over Regulation." *Congressional Quarterly Weekly Review* 41:501–508.

Pfiffner, James P. 1992. "The President and the Post Reform Congress." in *The Postreform Congress,* ed. Roger H. Davidson. New York, NY: St. Martin's Press.

Pressman, Jeffrey L. and Aaron Wildavsky. 1973. *Implementation*. Berkeley: University of California Press.

Rich, Spencer. 1991. "Medicaid Dispute Tentatively Settled: States' Schemes to Obtain Extra Federal Funding Would Be Curtailed," *Washington Post,* 12 November.

Rivlin, Alice. 1992. *Reviving the American Dream: The Economy, the State, and the Federal Government.* Washington D.C.: The Brookings Institution.

Rosenbaum, Sara. 1994a. "Medicaid Expansions and Access to Health Care." In *Medicaid Financing Crisis: Balancing , Responsibilities, Priorities, and Dollars,* ed. Diane Rowland, Judith Feder, and Alina Salganicoff. San Francisco: American Association for the Advancement of Science.

————. 1994b. "Principal Federal Medicaid Legislative Reforms 1981–1991." In *Medicaid Financing Crisis: Balancing , Responsibilities, Priorities, and Dollars,* ed. Diane Rowland, Judith Feder, and Alina Salganicoff. San Francisco: American Association for the Advancement of Science.

Rovner, Julie.1989. "Reconciliation Dominates Policy-Making Process." *Congressional Quarterly Weekly Review* 47:964–968.

Rowland, Diane. 1992. Interview with the author, November 15.

Rowland, Diane, Judith Feder, Alina Saiganicoff, eds.1993. *Medicaid Financing Crisis: Balancing Responsibilities, Priorities, and Dollars.* San Francisco: American Association for the Advancement of Science.

Sardell, Alice. 1991. "Child Health Policy in the U.S.: The Paradox Syndrome." In *Health Policy and the Disadvantaged,* ed. Lawrence D. Brown. London: Duke University Press.

Skocpol, Theda.1988. "the Limits of the New Deal System and the Roots of Contemporary Welfare Dilemmas." in *The Politics Of Social Policy in the United States,* ed. Margaret Weir, Ann Shola Orloff, and Theda Skocpol. Princeton, NJ.:Princeton University.

Schick, Allen. 1990. *The Capacity To Budget.* Washington D.C.: Urban Institute.

————. 1995. *The Federal Budget.* Washington D.C. The Brookings Institute.

Schlesinger, Mark and Karl Kronebusch. 1990. "The Failure of Prenatal Care Policy for the Poor." *Health Affairs* 4: 91–111.

Schneider, Saundra. 1988. "Intergovernmental Influences on Medicaid Program Expenditures." *Public Administration Review* 48:756–763.

Sinclair, Barbara. 1989. "House Majority Party Leadership in the Late 1980s" In *Congress Reconsidered,* 4th ed., ed. Lawrence C. Dodd and Bruce I. Oppenheimer.Washington D.C.: Congressional Quarterly.

Slessarev, Helene.1988. "Racial Tensions and Institutional Support: Social Programs During a Period of Retrenchment." In *The Politics of Social*

Policy in the United States, ed. Margaret Weir, Ann Shola Orloff and Theda Skocpol. Princeton, NJ: Princeton University.

Smith, Steven. 1989. "Taking it to the Floor." in *Congress Reconsidered.* 4th ed., ed. Lawrence C. Dodd and Bruce L. Oppenheimer. Washington, D.C.: Congressional Quarterly.

Smith, Steven and Christopher J. Deering. 1990. *Committees in Congress.* 2d ed. Washington, D.C.: Congressional Quarterly.

Stein, Robert M. and Kenneth N. Bickers. 1994. "Congressional Elections and the Pork Barrel." *Journal of Politics* 56:377–399.

Stevens, Robert and Rosemary Stevens. 1974. *Welfare Medicine in America: A Case Study of Medicaid.* New York: The Free Press.

Stone, Deborah A. 1991. "State Innovation in Health Policy." Presented at Ford Foundation Conference on *The Fundamental Questions of Innovation,* May 3–4 at Duke University.

Surles, Richard C. et al. 1992."Case Management: Strategies for Systems Change." *Health Affairs* 11(1):151–163.

Tiebout, C.M. 1956. "A Pure theory of local expenditures." *Journal of Political Economy* 6:416–424.

Thompson, Frank. 1981. *Health Policy and the Politics and Implementation.* Cambridge, MA: Massachusettes Institute of Technology.

Thurber, James A. 1992. "New Rules for an Old Game: Zero-Sum Budgeting in the Post-Reform Congress." in *The Postreform Congress,* ed. Roger H. Davidson. New York, NY: St. Martin's.

Torres-Gil, Fernando. 1989. "The Politics of Catastrophic and Long-Term Care Coverage." *Journal of Aging and Social Policy* 12:61–86.

U.S. Congressional Budget Office. 1992. *Factors Contributing to Growth of the Medicaid Program.* Staff Memorandum. May.

U.S. Department of Health and Human Services. 1993. *Annual Statistical Supplement, 1993 to the Social Security Bulletin.* Document No. 993. Washington, D.C., August.

U.S. Department of Health and Human Services. 1993. *Health Care Financing Review: 1992 Medicare and Medicaid Annual Statistical Supplement.* Health Care Financing Administration. Baltimore, Md. October.

U.S. Department of Health and Human Services. 1995. *Health Care Financing Review: Medicare and Medicaid Statistical Supplement.* Health Care Financing Administration. Baltimore, Md. February.

U.S. House.1988. Committee on Energy and Commerce. Subcommittee on Health and the Environment. *Medicaid Source Book: Background Data and Analysis.* Report Prepared by the Congressional Research Service. 100th Cong., 2d sess. Committee Print 100–AA.

U.S. House. 1991. Committee on Energy and Commerce. *Medicaid Program Investigation: Hearings before the Subcommittee on Oversight and Investigations,* 102d Cong., 1st sess.

U.S. House. 1991. Committee on Energy and Commerce. *State Financing of Medicaid: Hearings before the Subcommittee on Health and the Environment,* 102d Cong., 1st sess., September 30, October 16.

U.S. House. 1993. Committee on Energy and Commerce. Subcommittee on Health and the Environment. *Medicaid Source Book: Background Data and Analysis (1993 Update).* Report Prepared by the Congressional Research Service. 103rd Cong., 1st sess. Committee Print 103–A.

U.S. House. 1990. Committee on Government Operations. *Medicaid Funding Crisis: Hearing before the Human Resources and Intergovernmental Relations Subcommittee,* 101sst Cong., 2d sess., December 7.

U.S. House. 1992. Committee on Ways and Means. *Overview of Entitlement Programs: 1992 Green Book.* 102d Cong., 2d sess., Committee Print WMCP: 102–44, 15 May.

U.S. Senate. 1969. Committee on Finance. *Medicare and Medicaid: Hearings before the Committee on Finance,* 91st Cong., 1st sess., 1–2 July.

U.S. Senate. 1970. Committee on Finance. *Medicare and Medicaid: Hearings before the Committee on Finance, Parts I and II,* 91st Cong., 2d sess.

U.S. Senate. 1970. Committee on Finance. *Medicare and Medicaid, Problems Issues, and Alternatives,* 91st Congr., 1st sess. Committee Print. 9 February.

U.S. Senate. 1989. Committee on Finance. *Health Care Coverage for Children: Hearing before the Committee on Finance,* 101st Congr., 1st sess. 20 June.

U.S. Senate. 1991. Committee on Finance. *HCFA Regulation Restricting Use of Medicaid Provider Donations and Taxes: Hearing before Committee on Finance,* 102d Cong., 1st sess., November 19.

Van Horn, Carl E., ed.1993. *The State of the States.* Washington, D.C.: Congressional Quarterly.

Verdier, James M. 1993. "State Provider Assessments to Fund Medicaid-- Figuring the Political Cost," *State Tax Notes.* :523–526.

Wade, Martcia and Stacey Berg. 1995. "Causes of Medicaid Expenditure Growth." *Health Care Financing Review* 16(3): 11–24.

Walker, David B. 1981. *Toward A Functioning Federalism.* Boston, MA.:Little, Brown and Company.

Waxman, Henry A. 1989. "Kids and Medicaid: Progress but Continuing Problems." *American Journal of Public Health* 79:1217–1218.

Weiner, Joshua M. and Jeannie Engel. 1991. *Improving Access to Health Services for Children and Pregnant Women.* Washington, D.C.: The Brookings Institution.

White, Joseph. 1995. "Budgeting and Health Policymaking." In *Intensive Care: How Congress Shapes Health Care.* ed. Thomas Mann and Norman Ornstein. Washington, D.C. :Brookings Institution.

Wildavsky, Aaron. 1992. *The New Politics of the Budgetary Process.* 2d ed. New York, NY: Harper Collins.

Wnuk, Christine. 1993. "Foiling Federal Mandates." *State Legislatures* 19(5):13.

Wright, Deil S. 1988. *Understanding Intergovernmental Relations.* 3d ed. Pacific Grove, Calif.:Brooks/Cole.

Zimmerman, Joseph F. and Sharon Lawrence. 1992. *Federal Statutory Preemption of State and Local Authority: History, Inventory, and Issues.* Washington, D.C.: U.S. Advisory Commission on Intergovernmental Relations.